The IBS Healing Plan

◆ ◆ ◆

Titles in the Positive Options for Health Series

Positive Options for Antiphospholipid Syndrome (APS) by Triona Holden

Positive Options for Children with Asthma by O. P. Jaggi, MD, PhD

Positive Options for Colorectal Cancer by Carol Ann Larson

Positive Options for Crohn's Disease by Joan Gomez, MD

Positive Options for Hiatus Hernia by Tom Smith, MD

Positive Options for Living with Lupus by Philippa Pigache

Positive Options for Living with Your Ostomy by Dr. Craig A. White

Positive Options for Polycystic Ovary Syndrome (PCOS)
by Christine Craggs-Hinton and Adam Balen, MD

Positive Options for Reflex Sympathetic Dystrophy (RSD)
by Elena Juris

Positive Options for Seasonal Affective Disorder (SAD)
by Fiona Marshall and Peter Cheevers

Positive Options for Sjögren's Syndrome by Sue Dyson

The IBS Healing Plan by Theresa Cheung

Ordering

Trade bookstores in the U.S. and Canada please contact:

Publishers Group West
1700 Fourth Street, Berkeley CA 94710
Phone: (800) 788-3123 Fax: (800) 351-5073

Hunter House books are available at bulk discounts for textbook
course adoptions; to qualifying community, health-care, and
government organizations; and for special promotions and fund-raising.
For details please contact:

Special Sales Department
Hunter House Inc., PO Box 2914, Alameda CA 94501-0914
Phone: (510) 865-5282 Fax: (510) 865-4295
E-mail: ordering@hunterhouse.com

Individuals can order our books from most bookstores, by calling
(800) 266-5592, or from our website at www.hunterhouse.com

Project Credits

Cover Design	Brian Dittmar Graphic Design
Book Production	John McKercher
Copy Editor	Jessica Bryan
Proofreader	John David Marion
Indexers	Robert and Cynthia Swanson
Acquisitions Editor	Jeanne Brondino
Editor	Alexandra Mummery
Senior Marketing Associate	Reina Santana
Publicity Assistant	Alexi Ueltzen
Rights Coordinator	Candace Groskreutz
Customer Service Manager	Christina Sverdrup
Order Fulfillment	Washul Lakdhon
Administrator	Theresa Nelson
Computer Support	Peter Eichelberger
Publisher	Kiran S. Rana

The
IBS Healing Plan

Natural Ways to Beat Your Symptoms

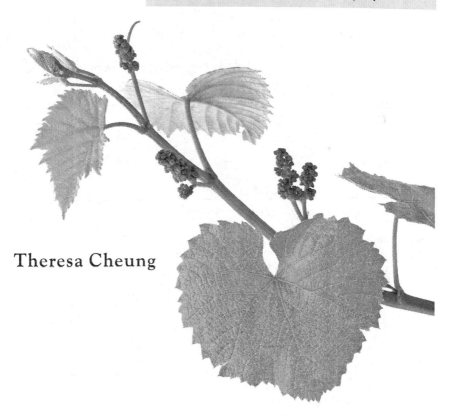

Theresa Cheung

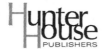
Hunter House
PUBLISHERS

Hunter House Inc., Publishers
PO Box 2914
Alameda CA 94501-0914

Library of Congress Cataloging-in-Publication Data

Francis-Cheung, Theresa.
The IBS healing plan : natural ways to beat your symptoms / Theresa Cheung.
p. cm. — (Positive options for health series)
Includes bibliographical references and index.
ISBN-13: 978-0-89793-507-4 (pbk.)
ISBN-10: 0-89793-507-1 (pbk.)
1. Irritable colon—Alternative treatment—Popular works. 2. Colon (Anat-
omy)—Diseases—Popular works.   I. Title.   II. Title: The irritable bowel
syndrome healing plan.
RC862.I77F73 2008
616.3'42—dc22   2008004913

Manufactured in the United States of America

9 8 7 6 5 4 3 2   First Edition   12 13 14 15 16

Contents

Introduction: Problems "Down There" 1

1. What Is IBS? 3
   Diagnosing Irritable Bowel Syndrome
   Symptoms of IBS
   Symptoms that Should Not Be Ascribed to IBS

2. What Causes IBS? 11
   Is IBS Inherited?
   IBS and Food Intolerance
   Is There a Neurochemical Imbalance in IBS?
   IBS and Analgesics
   The Role of Reproductive Hormones
   Mood and IBS
   Bacterial Overgrowth in the Small Intestine
   Leaky Gut Syndrome
   Your Early Warning Sign

3. Do You Have IBS? 19
   An IBS Questionnaire
   IBS Facts

4. Healing IBS with Diet 23
   Start with Healthy Eating
   Carbohydrates and IBS
   Protein and IBS
   Water and IBS
   Healthy Fats and IBS
   Adjusting Your Eating Habits
   The Seven Golden Rules of the IBS Diet
   Eating Out If You Have IBS
   Vegetarianism and IBS
   Weight Loss If You Have IBS

5. Healing IBS with Supplements 44
   Mineral Supplements
   Vitamin Supplements

Taking a Vitamin and Mineral Supplement
Herbal Healing
Digestive Aids
Finding Your Winning Formula

6. Healing IBS with Complementary Therapies 55
Healing with Acupuncture
Healing with Aromatherapy
Traditional Chinese Medicine (TCM)
Healing with Homeopathy
Healing with Hypnotherapy
Movement Therapy
Reflexology

7. Healing IBS with Stress Management 68
Techniques to Help Calm Your Mind and Your Colon
Behavioral Therapy
Exercise
Massage
Meditation
Music Therapy
Reiki
Relaxation
Visualization
Stress-Busters You Can Use Anytime, Anywhere
Get Your Z's

8. Working with Your Doctor 92
Over-the-Counter Medications for IBS
Prescription Medicines
Visiting Your Doctor
How Best to Proceed

9. A-to-Z of Specific Symptoms
and Natural Ways to Beat Them 100
Safety First
Abdominal Pain
Anxiety
Bloating
Constipation
Cyclical Symptoms of IBS
Depression/Low Mood
Diarrhea
Fatigue

Gas and Gurgling Stomach Noises
Headaches
Heartburn
Nausea

10. Living with IBS. 129
Fecal Incontinence
Covering Up Odors
Traveling by Plane, Car, or Train
Sex
Telling Other People
Helping Children and Teenagers Cope with IBS
Run, Don't Walk

References. 141

Resources 150

Further Reading 152

Index. 153

Important Note

The material in this book is intended to provide a review of information regarding irritable bowel syndrome. Every effort has been made to provide accurate and dependable information. The contents of this book have been compiled through professional research and in consultation with medical professionals. However, health-care professionals have differing opinions, and advances in medical and scientific research are made very quickly, so some of the information may become outdated.

Therefore, the publisher, authors, and editors, as well as the professionals quoted in the book, cannot be held responsible for any error, omission, or dated material. Nor can they be held responsible for the endorsement of any outside weight-loss agency. The authors and publisher assume no responsibility for any outcome of applying the information in this book in a program of self-care or under the care of a licensed practitioner. If you have questions concerning your nutrition or diet, or about the application of the information described in this book, consult a qualified health-care professional.

Introduction: Problems "Down There"

As far as discussions of health problems go, talking about irritable bowel syndrome, or IBS, is toward the bottom of the pile (pardon the pun). People don't seem to mind openly talking about diabetes, hypertension, even PMS, but mention bowel movements and folks get uneasy.

It's easy to understand why. How are you supposed to slip anecdotes like the following into normal conversation: "Sorry I didn't make it to the party yesterday, but I had the runs. I actually pooped myself in the car because I couldn't get to a restroom in time." What on earth would you expect someone to say in response? Or try telling your colleagues why it would not be a good idea for you to make a presentation to important clients: "I'd like to—really, I would—but chances are I'd be constipated for days beforehand, and then about half an hour before the meeting my colon would spasm and I'd have to cancel the meeting or excuse myself every few minutes for urgent trips to the restroom." It's also easy to understand why IBS gets so little media coverage. What journalist wants to get the latest scoop on bowel movements or discuss them on air? How would you persuade a celebrity to help raise public awareness, or attract sponsors to fund research?

Despite this reluctance to talk about it openly, irritable bowel syndrome affects as many as one in five people. That's a pretty serious statistic for an ailment described merely as "irritable." Yet in a society where bowel dysfunction is not considered a topic of polite conversation, it can be difficult to find help for IBS. In fact, according to the International Foundation for Functional Gastrointestinal Disorders, most people with IBS do not get the medical attention they need. If you think you may be one of these people, it's time to trust your gut, read this book, and come to grips with your discomfort about the topic.

The symptoms of IBS differ from person to person and can involve any of the following: intestinal spasm, constipation, diarrhea, hemorrhoids, and anal fissures (small tears in the anus caused by recurrent straining). Depending on how severe and frequent your symptoms are, IBS can either be a minor irritation or something that really interferes with your quality of life. Sadly, medical treatments for IBS don't always help, and some have side effects that are worse than the symptoms themselves. Some antidiarrheal medications can make people with IBS bloat like a beach ball and noisily expel gas all day, to the extent that even the diarrhea is easier to live with. The good news is that there are many effective natural treatments for IBS, and you'll find them clearly explained in this book.

Many people who have IBS try to overlook it, but IBS can't and shouldn't be ignored for long. *The IBS Healing Plan* confirms that IBS is real, and it shows you the many ways you can successfully deal with your symptoms, working with or without the help of your doctor. Because there is no wonder drug for IBS, people who have the condition often try all sorts of therapies for relief. This book sorts through the available remedies and outlines only the best and most effective ones. It presents a practical, holistic approach to IBS that will help you—or a loved one, if you are reading this book for someone else—leave the gas, pain, strain, and other problems "down there" behind for good.

Chapter 1

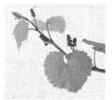

What Is IBS?

Jack, age 47

I was diagnosed with IBS about two years ago. Like most people with IBS, I have good days, bad days, and truly foul days.

About three months ago, I had a lunch meeting with a client from out of town. Things felt good, both business-wise and IBS-wise, and after lunch I headed back to my car to drive to my office. I began to feel the familiar IBS discomfort, but it was mild, and knowing that my office was only a ten-minute drive away, I thought it would be fine. It wasn't.

After five minutes in the car, the traffic came to an unexpected halt. I was at a standstill for about ten minutes, and I started to wish I had used the bathroom at the restaurant. I turned on the radio and heard that there had been an accident close by and there would be delays of up to thirty minutes. I knew I didn't have thirty minutes.

I decided to drive up the wrong side of the road so I could take a right turn that would take me to another street that led to my office. What I didn't know was that three cars behind me there was a police motorbike. The next thing I knew, there were red flashing lights in my rear view mirror. I pulled over and, squirming with embarrassment, told the policewoman I wouldn't normally break the law, but I have IBS and I had to find a bathroom. Sadly, she was not sympathetic and wrote out a ticket for an illegal turn. By the time she had handed it to me, it was too late. My pants were full and I had stained the car seat. I had no choice but to call the office and say I needed the rest of the day off.

Tracey, age 29

I became nervous about my bowel symptoms when a friend of mine was diagnosed with colon cancer. I don't know what symptoms she was having, but it got me very concerned. I went to my doctor and he did a thorough examination and asked me a lot of questions. He said that my symptoms were very similar to those of people who have irritable bowel syndrome. I asked him how he could be sure without doing any tests. He said that he couldn't be absolutely sure, but he was confident that I didn't have anything more serious. I told him I was really concerned, and that I would feel better if we did some tests. So now I am doing some home treatment and going in next week for some tests. Even if they don't show anything, I know that I will rest easier.

Linda, age 33

My daughter and I were renting a holiday cottage by the beach that had only one bathroom. She was in the bathroom when I had to go, so I had to use the cats' litter tray because I had forgotten to bring along my Porta Potty.

While on vacation I made so many trips to the bathroom that my daughter thought I had taken up residence there. At one point, while in the bathroom, I started to think about potty as an Olympic event, with ways of rolling the toilet paper and ways of wiping and toilet dismounting. Seriously, though, IBS has ruined my holiday, as it ruins most of my outings when I have to tear through places to get to the toilet.

Mark, age 18

I'll be eighteen years old in a few months, and since I began to suffer from IBS I've deteriorated very fast. The first time I got constipated it was so bad I had to go to the hospital to have suppositories administered. It was so embarrassing and really painful. It felt like I had years of waste inside of me that needed to come out but wouldn't. I was given strong painkillers and antisickness tablets to help prevent me from becoming sick every time I strained on the toilet.

When I went home, I did manage to go to the toilet, but I wasn't going much and it was painful. I always left the toilet weaker and more fragile than when I went in. Then the second attack came, which was worse than the first. I hadn't been able to go for a week and the cramping was excruciating. I had no energy to go back to the hospital again. I had no choice either. Off I went and had the same treatment as before. I had an interview scheduled in a few weeks for a job I really wanted, but how can I work when I get sudden attacks of IBS?

I'm scared of taking drugs. In fact, I'm scared of everything, even going out of the house. I don't know how to deal with it anymore; it's so embarrassing. And I have no idea why this has happened to me—why don't any of my friends who eat junk all day long have this problem?

If these IBS stories strike a chord with you, the chances are you have IBS or know someone who does. But what exactly is IBS?

One of the most important weapons in your battle against IBS— also called *spastic colon* or *mucous colitis*—is information. You need to know the enemy. Fortunately, over the past few years a great deal of new information regarding the brain–gut interaction that results in IBS has surfaced, and new discoveries concerning its nature and treatment are being made all the time.

If you're suffering from IBS, you're certainly not alone. IBS is estimated to affect 15–20 percent of people, and half of them have never consulted a doctor concerning their symptoms. Despite this, IBS is still the condition most frequently seen by gastroenterologists, and it's one of the top ten diagnoses in the United States. It is also, incredibly, the second leading cause of worker absenteeism (behind only the common cold). These are pretty amazing statistics for a condition that some people have never even heard of or regard as a very minor ailment.

Interestingly, because IBS is a "functional" condition, you can't actually be tested for it. Rather, it is determined by a diagnosis of exclusion. This is because there are no structural, inflammatory, biochemical, or infectious abnormalities present in IBS. In other words, when people with IBS are examined by doctors, no physical problem can be found. So, are you just imagining your symptoms? No—you absolutely are not! A functional disorder simply means that the problem is an altered physiological function (that is, the way your body works), rather than something that has an identifiable origin. In other words, although an IBS attack and its resulting symptoms are clearly visible as physical manifestations, the underlying cause behind these symptoms is not. Put another way, the root cause of the problem cannot yet be identified by yielding a positive result from any existing medical tests. So what then, precisely, is wrong with the way your body works if you have IBS?

IBS is indisputably a physical problem. Simply put, the brain–digestive system interaction of people with IBS influences their bowel pain perception and motility. The processing of pain information within the central nervous system varies between people who have IBS, and those who do not have the condition, with the result that the former group can experience even normal gastrointestinal (GI) contractions as painful. The interactions between the brain, central nervous system, and GI system in people with IBS do not function properly. People with IBS have colons that react to stimuli that do not affect normal colons, and their reactions are much more severe. The end result is heightened pain sensitivity and abnormal gut motility in the form of irregular or increased GI muscle contractions. This gut overreaction and altered pain perception cause the symptoms that characterize IBS.

To fully understand IBS, it's also important to recognize what it is *not*. IBS is not a form of bowel cancer or an inflammatory disease, such as Crohn's or celiac disease (although it can be secondary to these), nor is it a condition that leads to other life-threatening illnesses. Although IBS is still a complex functional disorder, it merely relates to a set of symptoms that fail to indicate disease in diagnostic tests, including lower abdominal cramping, pain, bloating, gas, diarrhea and constipation, vomiting, mucus in the stools, and a full bowel sensation after even a small meal.

In conclusion, although medical researchers aren't exactly sure what IBS is, they know it equates to bowel discomfort and irritation that can either send you running to the bathroom faster than the speed of light or desperately reaching for a laxative. Like an unannounced visitor who drops in when you're just about to go out, or the annoying caller who won't let you off the phone, IBS comes calling whenever and wherever it likes.

Diagnosing Irritable Bowel Syndrome

According to the International Foundation for Functional Gastrointestinal Disorders (IFFGD), clinical IBS is characterized by at least twelve weeks during a twelve-month period during which a person experiences abdominal pain or discomfort and recurrent diarrhea and/or constipation—conditions that should always prompt a visit to the doctor to rule out other causes.

As we have seen, IBS is diagnosed by its symptoms, not by a particular medical test. This is because, as mentioned above, an irritable bowel is a normal, healthy bowel that for some reason does not function properly. Distressing as a diagnosis of IBS is, never forget that it does not lead to bowel cancer or other serious bowel disorders, such as colitis and Crohn's disease.

Symptoms of IBS

The symptoms of IBS depend on which parts of the gut are involved. Some people experience problems in only one part of the gut, others in several. Symptoms are unpredictable and can also vary over time. For example, for several months, weeks, or days you might suffer from bouts of diarrhea, and then for several months, weeks, or days you might suffer from constipation. Listed below are typical symptoms and the areas of the digestive system involved.

Symptoms Relating to the Esophagus

♦ A sensation like a golf ball in the throat between meals that does not interfere with swallowing

♦ Heartburn—a burning pain that is often felt behind the breastbone

♦ Painful swallowing, but without the hold-up of food

Symptoms Relating to the Stomach

♦ Non-ulcer dyspepsia (symptoms suggestive of a stomach or duodenal ulcer that has not been confirmed on investigation)

♦ Feeling full after small meals, which might eventually cause one to not be able to finish a meal

♦ Abdominal bloating after meals

Symptoms Relating to the Small Bowel

♦ Increased gurgling noises that might be loud enough to cause social embarrassment

♦ Abdominal bloating that can be so severe that women describe themselves as looking pregnant

♦ Generalized abdominal tenderness associated with bloating

♦ Abdominal bloating of both types that usually subsides overnight and returns the following day

Symptoms Relating to the Large Bowel

♦ Abdominal bloating of both types (see above list), which usually subsides overnight and returns the following day

♦ Right-sided abdominal pain, either low or tucked up under the right-hand ribs, that is not always relieved on opening of the bowels

- Pain tucked up under the left-side ribs that, when extreme, may enter the left armpit

- Variable and erratic bowel habits alternating between constipation and diarrhea

- Increased gastro-colic reflex, which is an awakening of the reflex in which food in the stomach stimulates colonic activity, resulting in the need to empty the bowels

- Severe, short, stabbing pains in the rectum, a condition called *proctalgia fugax*

Other Symptoms Associated with IBS

- Headaches

- In women, left-sided abdominal pain during sex

- Passing urine more frequently

- Fatigue and tiredness

- Sleep disturbance

- Loss of appetite

- Nausea

- Depressive symptoms in about one-third of the people who have IBS

- Anxiety and stress-related symptoms that may interact with gut symptoms

Doctors look for a specific pattern of symptoms when making a diagnosis, and if you have at least three of the five most common symptoms—abdominal pain, infrequency of bowel movements with bouts of diarrhea and/or constipation, mucus in the stools, a sensation of incomplete emptying of the rectum after going to the bathroom, and a bloated or distended feeling in the abdomen—then you meet the criteria for a diagnosis of IBS.

Symptoms that Should Not Be Ascribed to IBS

Because IBS can mimic so many other intestinal disorders, it's important to identify the symptoms that are not connected to IBS but that can easily be confused with IBS. If any of the following occur, you should see your doctor immediately:

- Difficulty in swallowing and when food gets stuck in the throat

- Indigestion-type pain that wakes you up during the night

- Abdominal bloating that does not get better overnight

- Significant and unexplained weight loss

- Bleeding from the rectum

- Chronic, painless diarrhea

This list is not comprehensive. If you are experiencing other symptoms, you should seek further advice.

(*Note:* Although IBS never causes bowel cancer or bowel damage, first-time symptoms of what seem to be IBS in a person, especially people over the age of forty, should be assessed by a doctor.)

Chapter 2

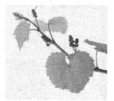

What Causes IBS?

Sally, age 26

I get really frustrated when doctors minimize the impact that IBS has had on my life. Just because my doctor can't find anything on the lab tests and has no idea what is causing my problems, he tells me it's not worth worrying about. That's easy for him to say. IBS has ruined my social life. I can't even enjoy dinner with my boyfriend without worrying about ending up looking and feeling like a hot-air balloon at the end of the night.

Interestingly, the origins of IBS might really be in our brains, and not in our bowels. Given that for many years people with IBS were told dismissively that their problem was "all in their heads," it's ironic that, in the end, this might be factually correct. The underlying problem might well be in your brain, but this does *not* mean it is in your imagination.

Although research is ongoing, no one really knows yet exactly why some people develop IBS and others don't. A great deal of research has been devoted to discovering the causes, especially the gut and brain interaction, but although we have learned a lot, crucial questions remain unanswered.

For many years, researchers thought that IBS was caused by poorly coordinated muscular contractions in the gut, but studies have shown that although people with IBS do sometimes have this problem, it does not always occur. As a result, doctors and medical researchers have had to look elsewhere for other possible causes. Here's a round-up of the latest research conclusions.

Is IBS Inherited?

Often IBS seems to "run in the family," thus raising the possibility that IBS is an inherited condition. When confronted with such questions of "nature versus nurture," investigators often study identical twins who were raised apart; however, these studies are certainly not definitive, because the number of twins with GI problems who are available for study is obviously limited. Talley and his colleagues in Australia reported on the GI symptoms experienced by 437 pairs of twins with abdominal pain, and they found that bowel symptoms occurred in both twins to a greater degree than would be expected by chance alone, but it was far from 100 percent. Thus, they concluded that although genetics might, in part, explain the occurrence of IBS, other environmental factors must be involved.

IBS and Food Intolerance

Studies show that between 33 and 66 percent of people with IBS report having one or more food intolerances. The most common culprits are dairy products (40–44 percent) and grains (40–60 percent). The fact that some but not all of the people with IBS report food intolerances suggests that it is not the primary cause. (If you think certain foods might be causing or triggering symptoms, be sure to read the dietary advice in Chapter 4, "Healing IBS with Diet.")

Is There a Neurochemical Imbalance in IBS?

Interaction or communication between the brain and the gut occurs via nerves that send neurotransmitter signals. An imbalance between two of these neurotransmitters, serotonin and norepinephrine, is implicated in IBS. Constipation might result when levels of norepinephrine increase, causing a reduction in serotonin levels and the inhibition of another neurotransmitter, acetylcholine. Conversely, diarrhea can occur when increased serotonin inhibits norepinephrine and causes levels of acetylcholine to increase. This means that people with IBS have an imbalance in their nervous system that can lead to the fluctuating bowel symptoms of constipation and diarrhea. Research on nerve function is spearheading IBS research at the present time, and there is evidence to suggest that there might well be differences in the brains of people with IBS and in the way they experience bowel movements.

IBS and Analgesics

The use of acetaminophen, a common pain-relieving medication, is associated with diarrhea-predominant IBS. Its action might be due to an imbalance in the neurotransmitter serotonin. Since acetaminophen can cause elevated levels of the serotonin by-product 5-HIAA in the urine, it is possible that acetaminophen somehow interferes with serotonin metabolism. Plasma serotonin levels have, indeed, been shown to be elevated after eating in people with diarrhea-predominant IBS. Clinically, a drug that blocks the 5-HT3 serotonin receptor (5-HT3 receptor antagonist) provides effective relief for women with diarrhea-predominant IBS.

The Role of Reproductive Hormones

IBS occurs more than twice as frequently in women than in men and tends to follow a cyclical pattern, with aggravation during the post-ovulatory (progesterone-dominant) and premenstrual phases of the menstrual cycle. Progesterone is known to delay gastric emptying and cause constipation. Constipation with straining and the frequent passage of hard stools is a more prevalent IBS manifestation in women, especially during the post-ovulatory or PMS phase, which begins about fourteen days before a period. At the end of the post-ovulatory phase, the sudden withdrawal of progesterone that occurs with the start of the premenstrual phase can trigger increased bowel activity. Women frequently report loose stools and diarrhea before or with the onset of menstruation. In contrast to progesterone, estrogen has not been associated with exacerbations of IBS symptoms.

In one study, high levels of the reproductive hormone luteinizing hormone (LH) were found in women with IBS. Drugs that decreased LH levels, and consequently suppressed ovarian production of estrogen and progesterone, resulted in significantly improved IBS symptoms. LH is a reproductive hormone responsible for the production of testosterone in males and estrogen and progesterone in women. In men, the opposite result was found: low LH and low testosterone (male hormone) tended to be associated with IBS symptoms. High LH, therefore, appears to cause exacerbations in women by stimulating progesterone and estrogen, yet it appears to have a protective effect in men.

In addition to progesterone levels in women, prostaglandins E2 and F2 alpha also increase during the premenstrual phase. Since they are powerful stimulants of bowel contractions, it is possible that women with IBS have an exaggerated response to these prostaglandins. (If you are a woman and suffer from increased bloating and constipation the week before your period, and looser bowel movements during your period, the advice in Chapter 9 about cycling symptoms of IBS and PMS will prove helpful.)

Mood and IBS

Anxiety, hostile feelings, sadness, depression, and sleep disturbance are associated with IBS. Adverse life events, such as a family death, marital stress, financial difficulties, and especially physical and sexual abuse, have also been reported more frequently in people with IBS than in the general population. However, it is possible that people with IBS from these social or psychological backgrounds are more likely to seek medical treatment or participate in research studies, and therefore these backgrounds become more identifiable.

The impact of stress on bowel motility and pain was explored in one study through the administration of corticotrophin-releasing factor (CRF), a hormone released in the body during stress. CRF increases motility of the descending colon and can induce abdominal pain. The researchers found that people with IBS had greater colonic motility and more abdominal pain after receiving CRF than controls.

Bacterial Overgrowth in the Small Intestine

An overgrowth of bacteria in the small intestine, an area that is normally relatively free of bacteria, is being recognized as important in the development of IBS. When these bacteria are present in the small intestine, excessive gas, bloating, abdominal distension and pain, and altered gut motility, can result.

The causes of small-intestine bacterial overgrowth include decreased gastric acid secretion (possibly due to natural ageing, stomach ulcers, and colonization by *Helicobacter pylori* bacteria), decreased bile flow, or decreased pancreatic enzymes, which cause poor absorption of carbohydrates, fats, and proteins. The resulting undigested and unabsorbed carbohydrates in the small intestine and colon cause excess fermentation and encourage growth of unwanted bacterial species. An abundance of gas is produced, as well as short-chain organic acids, such as lactic acid, which can damage the mucous lining of the intestines and further contribute to poor absorption of carbohydrates. In addition, putrefaction of proteins in the small intestine produces substances called *vasoactive amines* that can affect intestinal muscles.

There is mounting evidence that for some people with IBS the condition is precipitated by some type of severe attack on the gut —dysentery, food poisoning, intestinal flu, abdominal surgery, even pregnancy. The theory goes that even after full physical recovery from these traumatic events, the nerves within the gut retain a "memory" of the insult and remain hypersensitive to further stimulation, as well as prone to excess bacteria accumulation and subsequent overreaction.

Leaky Gut Syndrome

Some experts believe that IBS is associated with a condition known as *leaky gut syndrome*, sometimes called *gut dysbiosis*. We all have bacteria in our guts that is vital for good digestion and the health of the intestines. Unfortunately, the body often becomes infested with bad bacteria, and when this happens, the levels of good bacteria are lowered and digestion is compromised. When there is an overgrowth of bad versus good bacteria in your gut, leaky gut syndrome occurs.

Even though research has not yet confirmed a firm link between leaky gut syndrome and IBS, to have this condition is bad news for a number of reasons:

- With digestion compromised, leaky gut syndrome can trigger stomach upsets, bloating, constipation, and diarrhea—all symptoms of IBS.

- It produces toxins that can damage the intestinal walls and prevents good bacteria from producing the healthy organic acids that support colon health.

- Your immune system needs nutritional backup to function effectively, so when digestion is compromised, immunity is compromised as well, making you more susceptible to other infections, viruses, and diseases.

- Good bacteria aid food digestion and the production of vitamins and minerals; however, leaky gut syndrome limits the productivity of good digestion and causes nutritional deficiencies. If you are not getting the nutrients you need from your food, you'll feel unwell and tired.

- The bad bacteria and the toxins they create can make your gut hyperpermeable and more likely to allow unwanted particles of undigested food into your bloodstream. This can cause your immune system to be on high alert all the time, as it does not recognize these foreign particles, which results in food allergies, mysterious aches and pains, inflammation, fatigue, dizziness, foggy mind, and poor concentration.

Stress is believed to be a trigger for leaky gut syndrome. Experts argue that we have a second, more primitive, "brain" located in the stomach area, because there is a large concentration of nerves in that area. We all get "butterflies" in our stomachs when we feel anxious, frightened, or stressed. Your stomach and intestines are very sensitive to stress, and when you feel stressed, digestion shuts down to help the body focus on preparing the flight-or-fight response. This means that food is only partially digested, leading to leaky gut syndrome and nutrient deficiency. If the stress is long term, in time, the body gradually becomes less able to produce stomach acid and digestive enzymes, because it has become deficient in the vitamins and minerals required to produce these enzymes. Thus, a vicious circle occurs.

Another trigger for leaky gut syndrome is thought to be a diet high in sugar, refined carbohydrates, and processed food, because this type of diet deprives the body of nutrients, compromises digestion, limits the productivity of good bacteria, and feeds bad bacteria in the gut. Unfortunately, the standard Western diet is high in refined carbohydrates and sugar, and low in fiber, protein, and fresh uncooked fruits and vegetables—a recipe for leaky gut, and, some might say, IBS symptoms.

Your Early Warning Sign

The possible causes for IBS outlined above offer fascinating insights into why some people get IBS and some don't, but none of them fully explain the condition, and there are still those who are exceptions to every theory and who are still patiently waiting for an explanation. Despite this, the work of researchers is invaluable, because it can lead to better ways to understand and manage the condition. For example, new medications have been developed to relieve specific conditions, and understanding that your gut can be prone to bacterial overgrowth might encourage you to find ways to maintain a healthy bowel lining through the use of probiotic supplements. Also, recognizing that stress and poor diet can be a trigger will help you avoid or find ways to manage stress and possible nutritional deficiencies.

Right now the best approach to understanding IBS is to think of it as an early warning sign that you should step back and take a look at your diet and lifestyle. By learning your own triggers you can take control of your symptoms and lead a more IBS-free life. Chapters 4 to 9 of this book will help you do just that, but before we launch into the IBS Healing Plan, let's first make sure that you—or someone you know, if you are reading this book to help another person—actually has IBS.

Chapter 3

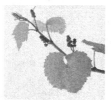

Do You Have IBS?

Take some time to answer the questions below and read the accompanying information, because your answers will help you to more precisely identify whether or not you have IBS.

An IBS Questionnaire

1. Do You Have Recurring Bouts of Abdominal Pain?

Recurring bouts of abdominal pain over a period of at least three months is the number-one symptom of IBS. This pain is often located in the bottom part of the abdomen below the belly button, but it can be felt all over the abdomen. The pain tends to decrease after a bowel movement. Although pain is common with IBS and does not indicate serious disease, you should still check with your doctor if the pain has recently appeared or is very severe.

2. Are Your Bowel Movements Abnormal?

Many people have one or two, even three, bowel movements a day, typically in the morning, and this is considered perfectly normal. If you have more than three or four bowel movements a day or less than one bowel movement a day, your bowel movements are considered abnormal. Bear in mind that we all have days or times in our lives when bowel movements are irregular for a few days, or even for a few weeks, due to a changes in routine (your bowels love routine!), such as a holiday or change of job or house, or a stressful event (for example, a divorce), but once you settle into a routine again your bowel movements should return to normal. If they don't, IBS could be the problem.

3. Have Your Bowel Movements Changed?

Another common symptom of IBS is irregular bowel movement patterns, interspersed with normal bowel function. For example, you could have irregular movements for one week out of every four.

4. Is There Mucus in Your Stools?

Many people worry that the presence of mucus in their stools indicates serious bowel disease, but mucus, without the presence of blood, is a common finding in people with IBS. Mucus is a normal by-product of the bowel and serves as a lubricant. More mucus than is necessary or normal is a symptom of IBS, just as a runny nose is a symptom of a cold.

5. Do You Suffer from Bloating or Abdominal Swelling?

Yet another unpleasant and common symptom of IBS, bloating is usually worse after eating and in the evening. If often disappears or improves overnight.

6. After a Bowel Movement, Do You Experience a Sensation of Incomplete Emptying of the Rectum?

You might strain unnecessarily after a bowel movement in an attempt to try and pass a stool. You have in fact completed your bowel movement, but the feeling of incomplete emptying is caused by the increased sensitivity of the gut. However, you should consult your doctor if you experience this persistently.

7. Do Other Nonbowel Symptoms Accompany Your IBS?

You might experience any one of the following nonbowel symptoms in addition to your IBS: heartburn, fatigue, urinary problems, migraines, and painful intercourse.

If you answered "yes" to at least three of the questions above and have experienced these symptoms for more than three months, the chances are you have IBS. If you feel that your symptoms do not exactly fit with IBS, then it is vital that you see your doctor immediately.

IBS Facts

Research studies have shown that the symptoms of IBS vary and can occur at any age. They most commonly start in the late teens or early adulthood, and most people start to experience symptoms before they are thirty years of age. In fact, if you are over forty and have encountered IBS symptoms for the first time, you should see your doctor, as the symptoms may have been caused by a recent intestinal infection.

As we learned in Chapters 1 and 2, IBS occurs because for some reason the bowel is more sensitive than usual and there are problems with coordination of the bowel. IBS also seems to be more common in women than in men, both in Europe and the United States. Curiously, in India more men report symptoms, although we don't know why this is.

Another distinguishing feature of IBS is that it does not always occur persistently. Symptoms can, and do, come and go over time, often triggered by dietary changes and stress.

The chances are you have looked into over-the-counter medications, such as laxatives, to relieve your symptoms, but the problem with long-term and frequent use of drugs is that they can actually make your symptoms worse because they aggravate your gut even more. No one drug can treat all the symptoms of IBS, and since

KEY STATISTICS

1. Irritable bowel syndrome is often confused with other conditions. It has been called by many names: *colitis, mucous colitis, spastic colon, spastic bowel,* and *functional bowel disease.* Most of these terms are inaccurate. *Colitis,* for instance, means inflammation of the large intestine (the colon), but IBS doesn't cause inflammation.

2. IBS symptoms affect up to 20 percent of the general population. It is the most common disorder diagnosed by gastroenterologists and is among the most common reported health disorders.

3. Women are two to three times more likely than men to suffer from IBS. Moreover, they seem to have more symptoms during their periods, suggesting that reproductive hormones play a role.

4. IBS is a chronic condition—you might develop it in your late twenties and have it for years, even for the rest of your life. Fortunately, the symptoms might come and go. The late twenties are the typical age of onset.

5. IBS can be triggered by stress, and flare-ups of symptoms are associated with major stressful life events in the majority of people with the condition. Studies indicate that some psychological treatments, such as cognitive behavioral therapy, can alleviate the abdominal pain and diarrhea associated with the syndrome.

the majority of people experience symptoms on and off throughout their lives, it would not be wise for these perfectly healthy individuals to take drugs for thirty or forty years, especially when most drugs have potential side effects. That's why it's best to avoid relying on drugs as much as possible and to use the natural healing techniques recommended in the chapters that follow.

Chapter 4

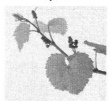

Healing IBS with Diet

Research makes it clear that diet plays a direct role in gut function (something that is instinctively obvious to people who have IBS), and symptoms are quite often triggered (not caused) by diet and dietary habits. Overeating, poor eating habits, and eating certain foods can cause trouble. Some types of food that typically irritate the colon include the following:

- Foods that contain caffeine, such as coffee, tea, chocolate, and soda
- Foods high in fat
- Spicy foods
- Alcohol
- Avocados
- Citrus fruits
- Corn
- Milk and diary products
- Sugar
- Wheat

If you think that any of these foods are a literal "pain in the colon" for you, the solution is simple: Stop eating them immediately and see if your symptoms improve after a week.

Jo, age 30

I went to my doctor two years ago and was diagnosed with IBS. He told me to switch to a bland diet. I didn't want to take drugs, so he put the focus on healing with food. As he suggested, I ate stacks of fiber-rich food, but it didn't help at all. I read some IBS books and went to some IBS websites on the Internet, and decided to cut out all dairy products, animal protein, sugar, and most fats. My symptoms got a little better, but I'd still have a few days every month when I was chained to the toilet. A friend of mine—who also has IBS—told me that chocolate might be making things worse for me. It was really tough to give up chocolate, because I adore it and have a few bars every day, but within a few days of giving up chocolate my cramps disappeared. It's depressing to have to give up something I adore, but there's no way I'd risk the pain and cramping again.

Start with Healthy Eating

If you've visited your doctor, it's probable that they have already suggested a change in diet, typically an increase in fiber, in the hope it will relieve your discomfort and normalize your bowel movements. Healthy eating is the first step to easing the discomfort of IBS. The second step is to adjust your eating habits based on what we know about the eating-related causes of irritable bowel. Many people with IBS jump immediately to the second step and skip the first, but laying the foundation with a healthy diet is crucial because your body needs adequate nutrition to function optimally and help you to cope with stress.

There's so much advice out there in magazines, books, and on the Internet that it can be hard to know exactly what constitutes a healthy diet. Basic good nutrition comes from a diet that—

- is balanced overall, with foods from all food groups, including lots of delicious fresh fruits, fresh vegetables, fresh whole grains, and fat-free or low-fat milk and milk products.

- is low in saturated fats, trans-fats, and cholesterol, and keeps total fat intake around 20–25 percent of calories, with most fats coming from sources of polyunsaturated and mono-unsaturated fatty acids, such as fish, nuts, seeds, and vegetable oils.

♦ includes a variety of whole foods, which are a good source of fiber; ideally, around 50 percent of total calories should be taken in the form of whole foods, including grains and fruits and vegetables. Whole grains can be a trigger food for some people with IBS, so refer to the advice below on soluble and insoluble fiber.

♦ includes a variety of fruits and vegetables. Eat at least five to seven servings of fruits and vegetables per day. They are an important source of vitamins, minerals, fiber, and phytochemicals, which provide disease-protective effects to the body.

♦ includes high-quality protein in the form of nuts, seeds, fish, lean meat, and whole grains; ideally around 20 percent of our calories should come from protein.

♦ has foods prepared with low levels of sodium (salt) because a high intake of sodium in the diet increases the risk of high blood pressure (aim for no more than about one teaspoonful of salt per day).

♦ includes plenty of fluids, ideally in the form of water (six to eight glasses a day is typically recommended) or juices.

The nutrients in food are fuel, and you need that fuel to feel well, digest your food efficiently, function normally, and cope with stress. Making sure your diet is healthy—and that you obtain adequate nutrition from a balanced intake of carbohydrates, proteins, and healthy fats, with at least six-to-eight glasses of water a day—is an essential foundation for good health, whether you have IBS or not.

Carbohydrates and IBS

When eaten, carbohydrates are broken down into glucose. We need glucose because it is the major fuel for the brain, muscles, and immune system. Complex carbohydrates (i.e., unrefined foods, such as grains, fruit, vegetables, nuts, and seeds) are by far the best way to get your carbohydrates, because they are packed with nutrients and are great for your digestion and energy levels. Refined carbohydrates (i.e., processed foods, such as cakes, sweets, ready meals, and white bread) flood the system with sugar as soon as they are eaten, providing a quick flash of energy followed by fatigue. In contrast, unrefined carbohydrates release their sugar slowly so that the blood sugar level stays in the normal range instead of fluctuating rapidly. When blood sugar is low we crave sweets and easily become angry or anxious, but when blood sugar levels are steady we can concentrate better and don't have food cravings. Another benefit of unrefined carbohydrates is that they are high in fiber; this boosts digestion, removes toxins, and encourages regular bowel movements.

Protein and IBS

Protein is the basic building block of all living cells; it makes up hormones, enzymes, antibodies, and immune cells. Adequate protein intake is essential for health and well-being. The constituents of protein are amino acids. There are eight of them that are vital to life, and they can be found in lean meat, fish, low-fat dairy, and produce, as well as in beans, lentils, nuts, and seeds. Amino acids perform essential functions. Some control memory, sleep, mood, energy levels, and how our digestive system functions. A poor diet can easily create an amino acid deficiency. Healthy forms of complete protein (i.e., those that contain all eight essential amino acids) include quinoa, tofu, fish, lean chicken, and combined pulses and grains.

Water and IBS

Water is the body's single most important nutrient. Almost all of the body's functions, including the immune system, rely on water. It carries nutrients to the cells; carries waste and toxins away from the cells and out of the body; maintains the body's temperature; and provides protection and cushioning for the joints and organs of the body as well as the skin. We lose water constantly through physiological processes, such as sweating, elimination, and breathing, and this water needs to be replenished. The body does not keep a reserve of water, as it does with other nutrients, so our need for water is continuous. Experts recommend that a healthy adult should drink around eight glasses of water per day. Sometimes we need more water because of accelerated water loss due to heat, excessive sweating, diarrhea, etc. Don't wait until you feel thirsty to drink water, because thirst is a sign of dehydration.

Avoid ice-cold foods and drinks on an empty stomach. Cold makes muscles contract, and your goal is to keep your stomach and the rest of your digestive system as calm as possible. Although you need to drink fresh water constantly throughout the day, you should limit the amount of water or other fluids you drink with your meals, because excess fluids can inhibit digestion.

Healthy Fats and IBS

Cold-pressed, unrefined nut or seed oils, such as flaxseed, walnut, or pumpkin seed oils, contain the essential fatty acids omega-6 linoleic acid and omega-3 alpha-linolenic acid. In the body, these fatty acids are converted into prostaglandins, which are essential for their inflammatory-reducing properties and the promotion of healthy colon function.

The best seeds and oils for essential fats are flax, linseeds, pumpkin, hemp, sunflower, safflower, sesame, corn, walnut, soybean, and wheat germ. Use the oil daily on salads or in other dishes. Note that the oil loses critical nutrients when heated, so make sure you consume it cold. Cold-water fish oils from salmon and mackerel are another good source for essential fatty acids. For best results, eat fish and a salad with a dressing of unrefined, cold-pressed sunflower or walnut oils. The fatty acid in fish helps to ensure the conversion of the oil's linoleic acid to colon-friendly prostaglandins.

Adjusting Your Eating Habits

Healthy eating is the first step. The second step is to start adjusting your eating habits according to the guidelines below. These food-related suggestions are really worth trying. They have worked for many people—but remember, we don't really know what causes IBS, so there is no "magic bullet" to cure it; what works for one person might not work for another.

1. Keep a Food Journal

Record everything you eat and drink for at least ten days and try to work out how your diet relates to your symptoms by comparing what you have eaten with severe IBS attacks. Write down everything you eat and drink, and every symptom you experience (such as abdominal pain, diarrhea, gas, bloating, and so on), how long it lasts, and how severe it is. Try to write down, too, how much you eat, where and how you eat, how long it takes you to eat your meal, and also what mood you are in when you eat. For example, did you eat a full plate of food? Did you eat on the move? Did you feel relaxed while you were eating? Becoming aware of which foods and eating habits can trigger attacks will help you avoid that food or situation and find alternatives. Bear in mind that it's normal to have contractions of the colon about thirty to sixty minutes after a meal. The box below offers some suggestions on how to keep a food journal.

HOW TO KEEP A FOOD JOURNAL

- Use a small notebook that you can carry with you and keep handy.
- Organize each page into columns. This can be done by using one page for each meal/snack, one page per day, or whatever works best for you (and the size of your notebook!).
  - The first column is "How much?" Estimate the size (inches), weight (ounces), volume (cups) or number (e.g., 5) of the food you eat.
  - The second column is "What kind?" What kind of food did you eat? Be very specific, and be sure to remember condiments and toppings, such as butter, salad dressings, mayonnaise, etc.
  - The third column is "Time." At what time of day did you eat the food?

(cont'd.)

- The fourth column is "Where?" Write down where you ate—in a restaurant, at the dining room table, over the sink, in your car, etc.
- The fifth column is "Who?" Fill in who you were eating with or whether you were alone.
- The sixth column is "Activity." Write down what you were doing while you ate. Were you working, driving, watching television, doing homework, etc.?
- The seventh column is "Mood." Take notes on how you were feeling while you were eating. Were you happy, sad, angry, stressed, etc.?
- The eighth, and probably the most important, column is "Symptoms." Write down any symptoms you might have experienced after you ate. Some examples might be diarrhea, stomach upset, bloating, gas, or heartburn.

- Be honest! It's important to report everything (even those potato chips you ate at 1:00 A.M.!).

- Update your records as you eat during the day. It can be difficult to remember everything you ate if you only make entries once each day.

- Be specific. The way a food was prepared or what it was served with can be important. For example, "roast potatoes" is a better description than just "potatoes."

- Stick with it! You might be amazed at how a simple food journal can help you and your doctor with your treatment.

2. Avoid IBS Trigger Foods

One of the fundamental principles behind healing IBS with diet is to avoid foods that trigger or irritate a spastic colon via the gastro-colic reflex, which occurs when food enters the stomach, and to eat foods that soothe and regulate the colon.

Please don't read this list and think you can never eat any of these trigger foods again. Although they are all IBS triggers, and some of them might need to be eliminated from your diet, others can still be eaten as long as you follow the advice outlined below on what and how you can eat if you have IBS. Try not to think of this as the beginning of a diet, but the beginning of a healthier way of eating.

Common IBS Triggers

♦ Red meat (minced beef, hamburgers, hot dogs, steaks, roast beef, pastrami, salami, bologna, pepperoni, corned beef, ham, bacon, sausage, pork chops, and anything else that comes from cows, pigs, sheep, goats, and deer, etc.).

♦ The dark meat and skin of poultry (skinless white meat is fine, as is seafood; try to buy organic turkey and chicken).

♦ Dairy products (cheese, butter, sour cream, cream cheese, milk, cream, half-and-half, ice cream, whipped cream, yogurt, and frozen yogurt). Even if you are not lactose intolerant, dairy products can be an IBS trigger food. It's not the lactose, but the high fat content of most dairy products that can cause symptoms. Even skimmed, semi-skimmed, and lactose-free dairy foods can trigger IBS attacks. In addition to fat and lactose, dairy products contain components, such as the proteins whey and casein, that can cause severe digestion problems.

♦ Saturated fat. The gut normally responds to food by contracting, and the strength of the response seems to be linked to the amount of saturated fat in the meal. So try to cut down on the saturated fat in your diet. Make sure that your milk is skimmed or semi-skimmed; cook with minimal fat by baking or steaming food rather than frying or roasting; and choose foods high in monosaturated fats, such as olive oil, canola oil, peanut oil, peanuts, cashews and almonds.

The following is a list of saturated, fat-rich foods to avoid:

– Dairy products	– Red meat
– Egg yolks	– Butter
– Peanut butter	– Chips and French fries
– Tartar sauce	– Salad dressings
– Onion rings	– Oil-based spreads
– Fried chicken	– Olives

– Croissants, pastries, biscuits, scones and doughnuts, and pie crust
– Nuts and nut butters
– Potato chips (unless they're baked)
– Corn chips and nachos (unless they're baked)
– Store-bought dried bananas (they're almost always deep-fried)
– Solid chocolate (baking cocoa powder is fine)
– Solid carob (carob powder is fine)
– Corn dogs (a kind of hot dog deep-fried in cornbread batter)
– Anything battered and deep-fried
– Anything skillet-fried in fat of any kind
– Shortening, margarine, mayonnaise, and Cool Whip
– Hidden sources of saturated fat can be found in crackers, pancakes, waffles, baked goods, and mashed potatoes.

The thought of giving up these foods might seem shocking at first, but if you give it a try you'll be surprised by how easy it can be, especially nowadays when there are so many fat-free products and healthy, tasty substitutes that let you cook and eat safely while still enjoying many of your favorite foods. And whenever you're tempted to indulge in a high-risk treat, remind yourself that it might not taste as scrumptious when it's followed by a vicious IBS attack.

GI Irritants

In addition to saturated fats, the following items can also be dangerous. If they trigger an attack, the solution is simple: Avoid them and find healthier, safer alternatives.

♦ *Coffee*, both regular and decaffeinated, contains an enzyme that is an extremely powerful GI tract irritant. Go cold turkey today and drink herbal teas instead. Coffee and tea also contain caffeine, which is a GI stimulant and should be avoided, especially in higher doses.

♦ *Chocolate, sweets, and cakes* are high in saturated fat. When you want something sweet, there are healthy alternatives. (See the display box below for alternatives.)

SWEET ALTERNATIVES

If you're craving sweets, your healthiest alternative is to eat fresh or dried fruits, such as apricots, apples, or pears. Fruit is power-packed with antioxidants and nutrients that can give you a natural energy boost.

- As long as you can tolerate dairy foods, unsweetened, low-fat, live yogurt mixed with fruit (or a spoonful of low-fat jam now and then) is a sweet, creamy, satisfying, nutritious, and light alternative to sugary, fatty cakes and desserts that will weigh you down.

- Instead of guzzling a soda loaded with sugar, additives, and calories, try a smoothie made from the juice of real fruits. Smoothies are scrumptious, sweet, and full of goodness.

- Try a bowl of hot oatmeal, flavored with a pinch of stevia or maple syrup. It will satisfy your sweet tooth, keep hunger at bay, and give you a comfort fix at the same time. Stevia is an herb that is 300 times sweeter than sugar, with negligible calories. Use it sparingly in cooking or for sprinkling on cereals and desserts.

- A small bar of good-quality dark chocolate is naturally rich in health-boosting flavonoids. When eaten in moderation, dark chocolate offers chocoholics a healthy, low-fat alternative to high-fat, high-sugar chocolate bars.

♦ *Alcohol* is a GI irritant and often triggers IBS attacks, especially when consumed on an empty stomach (although small amounts of alcohol used in cooking are fine). At the time of this writing, no studies have proven that alcohol either instigates or worsens IBS, but drinking has been proven to have significant effects on the digestive system as well as the rest of the body. Many people with IBS find that an occasional drink does not worsen their condition, but some discover (as with other foods and drinks through trial and error) that it does have a detrimental effect. Additionally, the effect of alcohol on the liver, the stomach, and overall health should be weighed against the positive effects, as well as the importance of social drinking and your quality of life.

♦ *Carbonation* in soda drinks, cola, and mineral water can cause bloating and cramps.

♦ *Artificial sweeteners*, particularly sorbitol, can trigger pain, cramps, gas, bloating, and diarrhea.

♦ *Artificial fats*, namely olestra (Olean), can cause abdominal cramping and diarrhea in people who don't even have IBS, so just imagine what it can do to you!

♦ MSG (monosodium glutamate) is a food additive that has been linked to many types of digestive upsets. It can be avoided by simply insisting that your food and take-out meals are MSG-free.

♦ Avoid *chewing gum*, because it will cause you to swallow excess air, which can trigger problems.

3. Supplement with Essential Fatty Acids (EFAs)

Although you should steer clear of saturated fats, healthy fats are essential and necessary, because your body—and in particular your heart—needs healthy fats in order to function, so you should never go on a totally fat-free diet. Instead, keep your fat intake to 20–25 percent of your total calories and make your fats count. As mentioned above in the "Healthy Fats" section, the fats you include in your diet should be monounsaturated and contain the essential fatty acids omega-3 and omega-6, so choose fat sources like olive oil, canola oil, avocados, finely ground nuts, fatty fish, and flax oil.

It's especially important to have a high intake of omega-3 and omega-6 because they create prostaglandins, which are hormone-like substances that help keep the cardiovascular, immune, nervous, and reproductive systems healthy. Although omega-3 fats contain more linolenic acid than omega-6 fats, both also contain important health-boosting substances. There are thousands of other reasons to make sure your diet is rich in omega oils, but in the case of IBS, eating plenty of cod, herring, mackerel, sardines, and salmon, or supplementing with flaxseed oil if you don't eat fish, can aid your digestion.

(Note: Because all fats, even heart-healthy choices, are still potential IBS triggers, please follow the dietary guidelines detailed in the "Watch How You Eat" section below.)

4. Fill Up on Soluble Fiber

Although it's best to reduce or completely eliminate saturated fats and GI irritants from your diet, there's another crucial component to eating safely to control IBS: understanding the difference between soluble and insoluble fiber. Soluble fiber can help relieve both constipation and diarrhea, but insoluble fiber can make diarrhea worse. People who suffer from diarrhea should increase the amount of fiber they get from soluble fiber by supplementing with oat bran or psyllium (natural vegetable fiber), which is available in over-the-counter supplements.

For many people with IBS, soluble fiber is the single most important dietary aid, but soluble fiber is not typically found in foods most people think of as "fiber," such as bran or raw leafy green vegetables. Soluble fiber is actually found in foods commonly thought of as "starches," although soluble fiber itself differs from starch because the chemical bonds that join its individual sugar units cannot be digested by enzymes in the human GI tract. In other words, soluble fiber slows the digestion of food, giving the body more time to digest and absorb nutrients.

Good sources of soluble fiber include the following:

– Rice	– Pasta and noodles
– Oatmeal	– Barley
– Rice cereals	– Flour tortillas
– Soy products	– Quinoa
– Corn meal	– Potatoes
– Carrots	– Yams

- Sweet potatoes
- Rutabagas
- Beets
- Mushrooms
- Bananas
- Mangoes
- Turnips
- Parsnips
- Squash and pumpkins
- Chestnuts
- Apple sauce
- Avocados (although they do have some fat)
- Fresh white breads, such as French or sourdough (not whole-wheat or whole-grain)
- Papayas (which also act as digestive aids that relieve gas and indigestion).

5. Eat Insoluble Fiber with Caution

Insoluble fiber foods, such as whole grains, figure strongly in a healthy diet, but if you have IBS they need to be eaten with caution because, like saturated fat, they can trigger symptoms. Unlike saturated fat, however, you cannot simply minimize your insoluble fiber intake, because this will leave you with nutritional deficiencies. The solution is to eat the following insoluble fiber foods with caution, and you'll be able to enjoy a wide variety of them in very healthy quantities without a problem:

- Wheat bran
- Granola
- Seeds
- Popcorn
- Melons
- Grapes and raisins
- Pineapple
- Celery
- Cauliflower
- Cucumbers
- Green beans
- Muesli
- Nuts
- Rhubarb
- Dates and prunes
- Cherries
- Sweet corn
- Broccoli
- Tomatoes
- Fresh herbs
- Whole-wheat flour, whole-wheat bread, whole-wheat cereals
- Apples (these are much safer when peeled)

- Beans and lentils (these are much safer if mashed or
  puréed)
- Berries (blueberries, strawberries, blackberries, cranberries,
  etc.)
- Peaches, nectarines, apricots, and pears (these are much
  safer when peeled)
- Oranges, grapefruits, lemons, and limes
- Greens (spinach, lettuce, kale, collards, watercress, etc.)
- Whole peas, snow peas, snap peas, and pea pods
- Bell peppers (these are safer when peeled and roasted)
- Onions, shallots, leeks, scallions, and garlic
- Cabbage, bok choy, and brussels sprouts
- Sprouted seeds (alfalfa, sunflower, radish, etc.)
- Whole grains, whole-grain breads, and whole-grain cereals

The secret is not to eliminate these foods completely, but to eat
them with a larger quantity of soluble fiber. For example, you can
stir-fry veggies into fried rice or blend fresh fruit into a smoothie to
drink after a breakfast bowl of oatmeal. In general, peeling, chop-
ping, cooking, and puréeing fruits, vegetables, and legumes will significantly minimize the impact of their insoluble fiber. It's also best
to avoid eating foods containing insoluble fiber on an empty stomach and to eat them cooked or made into soups and sauces rather
than whole and raw. Cook and blend beans and lentils into sauces,
dips, soups, or spreads. Finely grind nuts and incorporate them into
breads or cakes with white flour, which provides a safe soluble fiber
base. Eat bran and other whole grains in small quantities, accompa-
nied by soluble fiber. Raw fruit and green salads are best eaten at the
end of a meal high in soluble fiber, instead of at the beginning.

Problem Fruits and Vegetables
The following fruits and vegetables can be particularly troublesome
for people with IBS:

- *Sulphur-containing foods* (garlic, onions, leeks, broccoli,
  cauliflower, cabbage, asparagus, and brussels sprouts). In

addition to having high amounts of insoluble fiber, these foods also produce significant gas in the GI tract, which can trigger an attack. As with all other fruits and veggies, they are extremely nutritious foods and should not be eliminated from your diet, simply treated with caution.

♦ *Acidic foods* (citrus fruits, vinegars, and cooked tomatoes) should also be treated with caution, because their acidity can trigger symptoms. Once again, follow the rules for insoluble fiber and eat these foods in smaller quantities, incorporated with the consumption of foods high in soluble fiber—but make sure you eat them.

♦ *Fructose*, a fruit sugar found in honey and fruit juice, can cause gas, bloating, and diarrhea, so it is best to eat this in small amounts and to combine it with soluble fiber.

If you have days when almost everything you eat seems to trigger an attack, avoid insoluble-fiber foods completely and restrict your diet to soluble fiber foods, if only in order to give your stomach a rest.

6. Keep Your Fiber Intake below 30 Grams a Day

Some people are so enthusiastic about increasing their fiber intake that they take in way over the limit of 30 grams a day without realizing it. Ideally, you should balance your fiber intake from both soluble and insoluble fiber sources to between 22 and 28 grams a day. Fiber is helpful because it absorbs water from the intestines and keeps moisture in the stool, thus preventing constipation. Fiber also creates a bulking effect in your colon that can help prevent diarrhea and painful spasms. Unfortunately, there is a fine line between too much and too little fiber, and if you eat too much it can cause excessive bowel movements, bloating, and gas. However, don't let this steer you away from increasing your fiber intake. The only way to find out if fiber can help is to give it a try. Bear in mind that it's normal to experience some bloating and gas during the first few weeks of a fiber-rich diet, so stick with it for a week or two. If things don't improve, you need to ease up on the fiber and try a different approach.

7. Watch How You Eat

Diet can help or hurt people with IBS, based on how different foods physically affect your digestive system. However, it's not just what you eat that counts—it's also *how* you eat.

First of all, eating smaller meals throughout the day is important. Smaller meals are easier on your already stressed digestive system. Eating four to six small meals and snacks throughout the day will aid digestion and ease your symptoms. Snacking on small amounts of food throughout the day will keep you from getting ravenous and then over-eating, which can overload your digestive system and trigger an attack. Eating little and often, and never allowing more than three hours between a meal or snack, has another benefit; it allows you to treat yourself to the occasional indulgence. When your stomach is well stabilized by a recent intake of soluble fiber you can afford an occasional bar of chocolate or slice of cake.

Second, make sure you take your time when you eat and chew your food thoroughly. Eating quickly encourages you to swallow too much air, which can cause problems. Food that hits your stomach without being chewed properly can further stress your digestive system. The message is simple: Take your time when you eat.

Third, if you are addicted to junk food, fast food, or food that is highly processed and refined, and tend to rely on ready-prepared meals instead of home-cooked ones, this is going to play havoc with your digestive system. Try to stick with foods that are as natural as possible and prepare your meals from scratch as often as possible. This is nutritionally sound advice, whether you have IBS or not!

Finally, it goes without saying that gulping your food down quickly, eating on the move, and arguing or feeling anxious while you eat will play havoc with your digestive system. The calmer and happier you are when you eat, the more likely you are to digest your food well. (See Chapter 7, "Healing IBS with Stress Management.")

A TYPICAL MEAL PLAN FOR PEOPLE WITH IBS

Breakfast: A bowl of high-fiber, whole-wheat cereal, such as untoasted muesli or oatmeal, with fresh or canned fruit and reduced-fat milk or calcium-fortified soymilk and/or whole-wheat or whole-grain toast with minimal dab of margarine or jam. Herbal tea.

Lunch: Sandwiches made with whole-wheat bread and low-fat cheese, lean turkey, or canned fish, and a side salad. Canned or fresh fruit with low-fat yogurt. Water, herbal tea, or diluted juice.

Main evening meal: Lean grilled chicken with lemon juice and pepper, served with salad, boiled new potatoes, or a baked potato, and whole-grain bread.

Snacks: You can spread snacks throughout the day—fresh fruit, low-fat yogurt, low-fat wheat crackers with low-fat cheese, frozen yogurt, pretzels, whole-grain rice, whole-wheat toast, or low-fat bran muffin. Water, tea, or diluted juice.

The Seven Golden Rules of the IBS Diet

1. Eat soluble fiber whenever your stomach is empty, and make soluble-fiber foods the biggest part of every meal and snack.

2. Aim to eat 22–28 grams, but no more than 30 grams, of fiber a day.

3. Never eat saturated fat on an empty stomach or without an accompaniment of soluble fiber.

4. As much as possible, eliminate all red meat, dairy products, fried foods, egg yolks, coffee, soda, and alcohol from your diet.

5. Make sure you get enough essential fats (or EFAs) and healthy protein every day.

6. Eat little and often, and don't go more than three hours without a meal or snack.

7. Take time to savor and enjoy your food; chew your food thoroughly.

For healthy eating adjustments for specific symptoms, such as constipation and diarrhea, see Chapter 9, "A-to-Z of Specific Symptoms and Natural Ways to Beat Them."

Eating Out If You Have IBS

Eating out at restaurants or at social functions can be tough if you've got IBS. It is especially trying when you are dining with people you have a professional relationship with or hope to date, because they are not likely to know about your IBS. So how do you handle eating out without bringing attention to your problem?

Tips for Enjoyable Eating Out

Have a Plan of Attack
Before you leave for the restaurant, decide what you will eat and how much you will eat. If you're afraid that you will be hungry and tempted to eat something you shouldn't, have a safe snack before you leave. If you know where you're going, phone the restaurant beforehand and ask about the menu. Many restaurants and catering venues also have web pages that include their menus.

Check Out the Bathrooms First
Ask the host or hostess where the bathrooms are located before you sit down to eat, or right after being shown to your table. If your dining companions don't know about your health problems, you can use the excuse of wanting to wash your hands before dinner. This way you'll know where the facilities are located, and you can check to be sure they're clean and well stocked.

Skip the Cocktails
Alcoholic drinks might not be a good idea for people with IBS. Try sparkling water or a virgin cocktail instead.

Ask Your Server
Don't be afraid to ask your server how a food is prepared or whether it can be prepared in a lean way, rather than in a fried or creamy way.

Ask for tomato sauce rather than cream sauce and look for menu items that are prepared using low-fat cooking methods—baked, boiled, char-broiled, barbecued, stir-fried, poached, roasted, grilled, steamed, or braised. Always ask for your salad dressing on the side. For dessert, choose frozen yogurt, sorbet, or fruit salad.

Watch the Appetizers

Appetizers like mozzarella sticks, nachos, chicken fingers, and hot wings are all fatty, fried, or dairy-filled foods that might not be good to your colon. If everyone else is having an appetizer and you're feeling left out, have some soup instead or dig into the breadbasket.

Anticipate Any Awkward Questions

If someone asks why you are requesting a certain dish to be cooked in a particular way, you could mention your illness briefly, but if you prefer not to, "I'm on a diet" or "I stopped eating red meat and dairy products" are also common responses that aren't likely to raise more questions.

Vegetarianism and IBS

Laura, age 54, describes how a close examination of her diet helped her IBS: "I was placed on every kind of medication. Sometimes they worked in the short term, but sometimes they didn't work at all. The doctor finally suggested trying to alter my diet in cycles, and we discovered that eating meat was my problem. I became a vegetarian and no longer have constant problems. Sometimes I even go years without any pain at all. It's worth the effort you put into it when you finally feel better."

A well-planned vegetarian diet that includes plenty of healthy protein closely corresponds to healthy eating principles for IBS in terms of fat, carbohydrate, and fiber content. Vegetarian diets tend to be low in saturated fat and animal protein, and they generally contain sufficient fiber, characteristics that have been shown to be beneficial for IBS. The only danger for vegetarians is that their diet can become too high in fiber—that is, more than 30 grams a day.

This can result in a worsening of IBS symptoms, such as bloating, gas, abdominal pain, and diarrhea.

Weight Loss If You Have IBS

Can you lose weight when you are trying to keep your IBS symptoms under control with diet? The short answer to this question is "yes, absolutely!" The IBS diet guidelines given above are very compatible with weight loss because they are nutrient-rich, low-fat, plant-based, and incorporate plenty of fiber.

The common sense rules of regular meals, smaller meals, mindful eating, and regular physical activity are great guidelines for both digestive and overall health. More information about the amazing benefits of exercise (particularly if you've got IBS) is included in Chapter 7. If you're feeling daunted by trying to manage your IBS through diet and lose weight at the same time, the following case history might inspire you.

Lucy, age 42

To celebrate the New Year I decided to take my partner, Steve, on a combination business/pleasure trip to Paris, as it's such a beautiful city. When we got on the plane, however, I couldn't get the seatbelt around me, and I had to ask the skinny flight attendant for an extension. We had barely even gotten off the plane when I became ill. My stomach hurt so much that it made the rest of my body ache. I was bloated, nauseous, and had cold sweats. All I wanted to do was to break wind, but I couldn't. We had planned to have dinner that evening with some colleagues. We went, but I spent the entire evening leaving the table every few minutes to go sit on the toilet and cry. Each time I returned, the table would fall silent and all eyes would be on me out of concern. It was very embarrassing.

That was the "straw that broke the camel's back." I vowed to myself that I was going to do something about my weight and my IBS. I could not, would not, continue to live like this. Spending all my spare time on the toilet or on the couch in pain and never wanting to do anything was just too much.

I must admit, I was not eating properly. I would have espresso and pastries for breakfast, cheeseburger with chips or
fried chicken for lunch, an espresso Frappuccino on the way
home, pizza or other fast food for dinner, and who knows what
for snacks and dessert. I probably drank four to six cans of
Coke a day. When all was said and done, I was easily consuming 4,000 calories a day of garbage!

I went on the Internet and read some books, and I started
to learn about IBS and how food can both help and hinder. I
cleaned out the cupboards, donated foods that were not safe
or healthy to a local food bank, and stopped drinking caffeine.
Now I drink lots of water, tea, and the occasional sports drink.
(I do okay with sports drinks, but some people don't.) I've also
starting eating less, eating more frequently, and watching my
intake of saturated fat.

I started going to the gym after work for just fifteen to
twenty minutes. Slowly I increased the length of my workout to
thirty, forty, fifty, and then even to sixty+ minutes! My weight
loss wasn't dramatic at first, just one or two pounds a week, but
my doctor told me this was the safest and most healthy way
to lose weight and keep it off. He was right. By the end of the
year I was down to a size fourteen, and I haven't been that size
for years. My diet and lifestyle changes have added a good ten
years to my life, and I feel like I'm living again. I never feel hungry because the next snack or meal is only an hour or two away
and the food I'm eating is tasty and satisfying. I also have an
occasional bar of chocolate. Even my sex drive has increased. I
can't say enough about how very important it is to take charge
of your diet and get some kind of exercise! Even if it is just a
walk around the block every day, it's a start! I have only called
in sick to work for IBS-related issues once in the last year, and
it is wonderful to be able to walk around my neighborhood
without sweating and being out of breath or wondering where
the nearest bathroom is.

Chapter 5

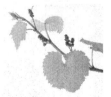

Healing IBS with Supplements

Many people with IBS have found supplements to be a better, safer, and more-effective option than drugs and medical treatments.

Sally, age 27

I tried taking digestive enzymes with acidophilus and found significant relief within three days. I am not afraid to eat now, but I still cannot eat very much refined sugar or high-fiber vegetables. I also have a cup or two per day of peppermint and chamomile tea. When I do have an episode, it occurs late in the day, but by the next morning I'm feeling back to normal.

Austin, age 44

I used to get bouts of painful diarrhea. Calcium carbonate, an over-the-counter supplement, has now helped me for more than two years. I take three tablets a day, one with each meal. The only side effect is that when you begin taking calcium you might have some gas or indigestion, but this usually goes away after taking a regular dose for a few days.

Laura, age 40

After about six months of a horrendously restrictive diet (ultra low-fat vegan with no raw veggies or fruit except bananas) and a lot of Metamucil [a fiber supplement], I managed to get my IBS partly under control. But if I deviated from the diet, the chronic diarrhea would come back. Someone I met told me that she had helped her IBS by taking a tablespoonful of freshly ground linseed with a glass of water or juice every morning. I thought it was another crackpot cure, but eventually I decided to try it. She told me that pre-ground linseed didn't work, because linseed starts to oxidize as soon as you grind it. She also said that whole linseed is no good either, because it cannot be digested properly. After years of IBS, in about two weeks it just went away. I cannot believe that I now have perfectly normal, regular bowel movements.

Recent surveys indicate that more than half of the people with IBS use supplements and alternative therapies (see Chapter 6) to seek relief. Listed below are the many types of supplements for IBS that can be very effective. In particular, soluble-fiber supplements, herbs that have beneficial effects on the GI tract (such as peppermint and fennel), probiotics, calcium and/or magnesium, and digestive enzymes are the most popular supplements that suggest proven benefit. Results are usually felt very quickly—sometimes even immediately.

There is no guarantee that any of the herbs or supplements discussed here will help you, but if you decide you want to experiment it's a good idea to make an appointment with an herbalist and/or nutritionist first, because, as stressed previously, your IBS symptoms and triggers are unique to you.

Note: If you are taking medication or are pregnant or hoping to get pregnant, you should consult your doctor before taking any supplements.

Mineral Supplements

If diarrhea is one of your symptoms, the chances are you will have lost many vital vitamins and minerals, and you may well need to use supplements to replace these lost vitamins and minerals in your system. Calcium is often the mineral most recommended by doctors, but other important minerals include magnesium and zinc.

Calcium

Most of us think of calcium as a mineral that is important for bones and teeth, but it has many other vital functions. Calcium is important for a healthy heart, normal nerve function, and muscle function. When taken with magnesium it provides the mechanism for muscle contraction and relaxation. Calcium also activates enzymes, allows the transport of nutrients through cell membranes, promotes cell division, and plays a role in iron utilization.

If you have IBS and are concerned about your calcium intake but can't tolerate dairy products, there are many other sources of calcium besides just milk and cheese. These sources include broccoli, spinach, turnip greens, tofu, yogurt, sardines and salmon with bones, calcium-fortified breads, calcium supplements, and some antacid tablets. For best absorption, calcium supplements should be taken with food, and doses should not exceed 500 milligrams at a time.

Magnesium

Magnesium deficiency is very common today because there is little magnesium in the earth's soil. The small amount of magnesium found in food is often lost during cooking and processing, and most of us simply do not eat enough magnesium-rich foods, such as whole grains, dark green vegetables, and nuts and seeds.

Calcium is important, but without magnesium, calcium cannot function. This is because magnesium works in synergy with calcium. If there is too much calcium and not enough magnesium, you can suffer from aches, pains, and fatigue. Because magnesium is crucial for carbohydrate metabolism, which creates energy, fatigue is in fact one of the first symptoms of magnesium deficiency. In terms of GI-tract function, calcium has a constipating effect, whereas magnesium acts as a laxative. As a result, calcium supplements can be truly beneficial for people with diarrhea-predominant IBS, and magnesium supplements can work wonders for IBS constipation.

Calcium/magnesium supplementation to keep your bowel function in balance is typically recommended in a 2:1 ratio of calcium to magnesium, because many people absorb magnesium more easily than calcium. Be careful that you do not exceed the recommended daily amounts of calcium (1,000 milligrams) and magnesium (400 milligrams).

Magnesium supplements come in many forms. Magnesium oxide has laxative effects that can be useful for constipation, but powdered forms of magnesium citrate are better for relieving diarrhea.

Zinc

Zinc is an essential trace mineral, which means that it must be obtained from the diet because the body cannot make enough. Low zinc levels have been reported in people with IBS. Zinc plays an important role in the immune system, which might explain why it is helpful in protecting against infections, such as colds. Zinc also plays a role in the regulation of appetite, stress levels, taste, and smell. Deficiencies in zinc can play a role in chronic diarrhea. The best food sources of zinc are legumes (especially lima beans, black-eyed peas, pinto beans, soybeans, and peanuts), miso, tofu, brewer's yeast, cooked greens, mushrooms, green beans, tahini, and pumpkin and sunflower seeds. Red meat and whole grains are also sources of zinc, but they are also potential irritants, so supplementation might be wise. Zinc sulphate is the most frequently used supplement, but it is also the least easily absorbed and might cause stomach upsets. Health-care providers usually prescribe 220 milligrams of zinc sulphate, which contains approximately 55 milligrams of elemental zinc. The more easily absorbed forms of zinc are zinc picolinate, zinc citrate, zinc acetate, zinc glycerate, and zinc monomethionine. If zinc sulphate causes stomach irritation, another form, such as zinc citrate, should be tried.

Vitamin Supplements

The main recommended vitamins for people with IBS are vitamins A, D, E, and K because they are not as easily absorbed as water-soluble vitamins are, and, like calcium and magnesium, they are likely to be drained from the body by diarrhea.

Vitamin A

Good food sources of vitamin A include dark green leafy vegetables, fruits, dairy foods, and eggs. Cod liver oil is the main supplement source.

Vitamin D

The main source of vitamin D is sunshine, and people who live in northern climates need extra vitamin D, which can be obtained from cod liver oil, vitamin D-fortified cereals, and fish oils.

Vitamin E

Vitamin E, like vitamin A, is a powerful antioxidant that protects the body from ageing and disease-promoting free radical damage. Food sources of vitamin E include vegetable oils, nuts, and green leafy vegetables.

Vitamin K

Vitamin K is responsible for blood clotting and is found in green leafy vegetables.

Taking a Vitamin
and Mineral Supplement

Diet should always be the foundation of good health, but if you have IBS and find it hard to eat a balanced diet, a combined vitamin and mineral supplement can provide important nutritional insurance. Research also indicates that food sensitivity that can trigger symptoms of IBS is more likely if you are lacking certain vitamins and minerals. Always choose a supplement that has as many vitamins and minerals as possible, in particular calcium, magnesium, zinc, and vitamins A, C, D, E, and K. Although there is no guarantee that this will improve your IBS, it will certainly help prevent nutritional deficiencies and improve your overall health. It might also help prevent some of the common health problems linked to vitamin and mineral deficiency, including: poor immunity, fatigue, PMS, poor wound healing, nose bleeds, dry skin, dull hair, gum disease, mouth ulcers, cracked lips, sore tongue, constipation, and fatigue.

Herbal Healing

Anise

Anise contains a type of oil that helps gastric juice production, and it can prevent and treat GI cramping. Anise can be used to treat both constipation and diarrhea because it helps to normalize bowel function. It is also a mild sedative and can ease stress and anxiety.

Artichoke Leaf Extract (ALE)

This extract might have potential for treating IBS. In a study evaluating the use of ALE in people with dyspepsia or indigestion, a small group was identified as having IBS. The severity of the symptoms in this group was reduced, which provided an overall favorable evaluation of the extract. As many as 96 percent of the participants claimed the artichoke leaf extract was well tolerated, and that it worked at least as well as the other therapies used for their symptoms.

Caraway

This is a very safe herb that can aid digestion because it increases the production of gastric juices and is a natural antibiotic. Researchers have found that several chemicals in caraway can help relax muscles in the intestines and eliminate the gas that causes pain and weight gain.

Cat's Claw

Cat's claw is a vine that grows in the rain forests of South America. In the villages of Peru, local medicine people have used cat's claw for hundreds of years to treat a wide variety of ailments, including stomach pain, ulcers, and other GI complaints. Modern research has found active ingredients in cat's claw that stimulate the immune system and have a possible antiviral effect. Cat's claw also neutralizes free radicals, the cell-damaging by-products of oxygen metabolism that contribute to inflammation. Cat's claw soothes irritated and inflamed tissues and helps to eliminate harmful organisms from the GI tract, making the herb potentially beneficial in IBS.

Chamomile

Research shows that chamomile can relieve GI stress by calming smooth muscle tissue, thereby relieving indigestion, gas, and bloating. The only possible side effect is an allergic reaction, because it's a member of the daisy family, which includes ragweed, a notorious allergen.

Evening Primrose

Evening primrose oil (EPO) is rich in GLA (gamma-linolenic acid), an essential fatty acid that reduces inflammation, supports immunity, and plays many other important roles. The human body can produce all but two types of the known fatty acids: the omega-3s and omega-6s. Both must be obtained through the diet or through the use of supplements. Obtaining a balance of these two fatty acids is essential. Essential fatty acids are needed for building cell membranes and are precursors for the production of hormones and prostaglandins. Modern diets tend to be lacking in quality sources of fatty acids.

Fennel

This licorice-flavored herb can help soothe the bowel by eliminating gas and bloating. It also helps increase the production of gastric juices, which can help digestion, normalize the contractions in the intestines, and relieve abdominal pain. It is a natural bowel relaxant because it contains dopamine. Research in Germany has shown that fennel is safe for daily use and can be effective for relieving abdominal pain, gas, and bloating.

Ginger

Ginger isn't just helpful for nausea—it can also ease indigestion and gastrointestinal cramps because it acts as a strong digestive enzyme.

Grapefruit Seed

Grapefruit seed extract is another remedy that might benefit people who have IBS because it helps prevent harmful organisms from populating the intestinal tract. Although the extract comes in liquid form, you can also eat the seed itself (although it is bitter!). Clinical and experimental studies indicate grapefruit seed extract has broad-spectrum antimicrobial properties. It also inhibits the growth of two ulcer-causing bacteria: *Helicobacter pylori* and *Campylobacter jejuni*. In one human study, grapefruit seed extract relieved constipation, gas, and abdominal distress after being used for four weeks.

Olive Leaf

Olive trees are widely cultivated throughout Mediterranean countries for their universally popular fruit. But olive trees have more to offer than just the olive and its delicious, healthful oil. The olive leaf has been used as a traditional medicine for treating health conditions, including malaria, infections, cardiovascular diseases, and for improving general well-being. *Oleuropein,* an active ingredient in olive leaf, shows promising antiviral properties. Lab studies have found that oleuropein stimulates the activity of immune cells, called *macrophages,* which serve as the body's "garbage collectors" to remove toxins and destroy foreign organisms.

Oregano

The oils in oregano can help relieve nausea, vomiting, diarrhea, and muscle cramps. They also increase gastric juice production and help eliminate gas and bloating.

Peppermint Oil

Peppermint is a favorite herb for relief of digestive problems, such as upset stomachs, gas, and colic in children. In Europe, peppermint oil is given routinely to people with IBS because of its relaxing, soothing effect. Peppermint oil helps relieve intestinal spasms, and its antispasmodic action has been demonstrated in laboratory animals. Peppermint oil relaxes the smooth muscle in the intestinal tract by acting as a mild "calcium channel blocker" to reduce muscle contractions. Many clinical trials have shown that enteric-coated peppermint oil relaxes the intestine and relieves pain in people with IBS. Enteric-coated pills are recommended because they dissolve better in the intestines, where they help relax the muscles and relieve pain.

Other herbs that might play a role in digestive and intestinal health include bitter orange peel, areca seed, and dandelion root. These are bitter herbs that can help stimulate gastric juices, and they also increase the production of bile, which helps to digest fats.

Digestive Aids

One of the best ways to boost your digestion is to chew your food properly, but you might also want to consider taking some digestive aids to make sure that no incompletely digested food reaches your large intestine and triggers IBS symptoms. Digestive enzymes are best taken in the middle or toward the end of a meal, and you should notice a decrease in bloating and flatulence within twenty-four hours of taking them. Typically, digestive enzymes contain various combinations of the following ingredients:

- Amylase: for digesting carbohydrates in the small intestine

- Betaine hydrochloric acid: for promoting digestion in the stomach

- Lipase: for fat digestion

◆ Papaya and bromelain: fruit sources for protein digestion

◆ Pepsin: for protein digestion in the stomach

◆ Peptidase: for protein digestion in the small intestine

Probiotics

Probiotic supplements are designed to help maintain a healthy population of *friendly* lactic acid-producing bacteria in the intestinal tract. (*Probiotic* means *for life*.) Also known as *friendly flora*, these bacteria help regulate elimination, support immunity in the gut, and keep "unfriendly" bacteria, such as *E. coli*, in check. As we learned in Chapter 2, it is theorized that people with IBS might not have enough of these good bacteria. This possibility was tested in a study of sixty people with IBS who took either a lactobacillus supplement or a placebo daily for four weeks. Compared to people on placebo, those taking the probiotic had far less intestinal gas. Twelve months later, overall GI function remained better in the people who had received the probiotic supplement.

You'll find probiotics in live yogurt, but since yogurt isn't always a good choice if you have IBS, you might want to try the capsule or powdered form. Probiotic supplements should be taken with food. Researchers believe there might be hundreds of different kinds of good bacteria in the gut and, not surprisingly, there are many different kinds of probiotic supplements available. In supplement form, look for doses in the billions of cells. The range of the most common probiotic, *Lactobacillus acidophilus*, is from one to ten billion active cells daily.

Soluble Fiber Supplements

Clinical studies have repeatedly proven the benefits of soluble fiber supplements for people with IBS. The USDA recommended minimum fiber intake for adults is 25 to 35 grams daily, and soluble fiber should account for one-third to one-half of this total amount. If you suffer from bouts of IBS constipation, you might want to take psyllium husk capsules or one to two tablespoonfuls of psyllium powder twice daily to maintain one or two bowel movements a day. The effectiveness of psyllium derives from a substance in the seed husk that swells to between eight and fourteen times its original volume when mixed with water. In the intestines, psyllium forms a laxative bulk that gently scrubs the bowel and absorbs toxins.

Finding Your Winning Formula

The supplements mentioned in this chapter have all been shown to be helpful to some people for treating the symptoms of IBS, and they might be helpful for you. Remember, though, that your IBS symptoms are as individual as you are, and what works for another person might not work for you. Keep experimenting with your diet and supplements until you find your own winning formula.

For more advice on supplements see Chapter 9, "A-to-Z of Specific Symptoms and Natural Ways to Beat Them."

◆ ◆ ◆

(Warning: If you are pregnant, on medication, or suffer from any medical condition other than IBS, be sure to seek medical advice before taking any herbs and supplements.)

Chapter 6

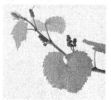

Healing IBS with Complementary Therapies

Complementary therapies can sometimes be of enormous help to people with IBS. Simon, for example, found relief using acupuncture, and Fiona found that homeopathy eased her symptoms.

Simon, age 31

I've suffered from IBS since I was 15 and have tried almost every supplement, complementary therapy, and medication there is. Some work better than others, but the only therapy I feel I can rely on 100 percent is acupuncture. When practiced by a trained, experienced, licensed practitioner of traditional Chinese medicine, acupuncture has helped relieve my very painful symptoms time and time again. I am also taking a prescribed Chinese herbal formula consisting of tiny, inexpensive pills. And eureka! No more IBS problems.

Fiona, age 30

I have suffered for several years from what the doctors have diagnosed as irritable bowel syndrome. My IBS came on very suddenly one evening, causing severe abdominal pain. The pain was so intense that I began to hyperventilate. My husband rushed me to the hospital, but the doctors could find nothing wrong with me. They gave me morphine for the pain and sent me home.

I made several visits to different doctors, and each one diagnosed IBS. They suggested I eliminate the foods that were causing the pain, get more exercise, and eliminate stress. They prescribed painkillers and muscle relaxants, and sent me home feeling hopeless. The painkillers caused drowsiness and constipation, and the muscle relaxants caused my heart to race. I knew that I couldn't continue to use them, and I really didn't want to anyway.

I wanted to find a natural way to combat this affliction. I took the doctors' advice and began walking to get my exercise. This seemed to help considerably, but I was unable to do it when I was in pain because it made the pain much worse. I also eliminated the foods that seemed to bother me, such as cabbage, broccoli, corn, soda pop, and ice cream. I began taking acidophilus, a glass of prune juice every morning, and a calcium supplement. This seemed to help relieve the pain and bouts of explosive diarrhea to some degree, but not enough.

My son, who is studying complementary medicine, suggested I try homeopathy. I wasn't sure, but by this time I was willing to give anything a try. I enjoyed the consultation because the homeopath didn't seem to be in a hurry like most of the doctors I've seen, and he wanted to know all about my diet and lifestyle. He urged me to continue the dietary measures I had already taken and to step up my stress management with some yoga. He also gave me an herbal remedy, and within days of taking it, I felt so much better. Within weeks I wasn't getting the cramps anymore, and within months I had my energy back. I still have to watch my stress levels and be careful about what I eat, but IBS isn't in control of my life anymore, I am.

The complementary therapies described in the remainder of this chapter have helped some people with IBS. Just as with traditional medicine and supplements for IBS, however, all treatments do not suit every person, so it is a matter of finding what works best for you. Remember, too, that your winning formula might not be a

single approach, but rather a combination of approaches: diet, supplements, complementary therapies, stress management, and consultation with your doctor.

◆ ◆ ◆

(*Warning: If you are pregnant, on medication, or suffer from any medical condition other than IBS, be sure to seek medical advice first before
experimenting with homeopathy, Chinese herbal medicine, and aromatherapy.*)

Healing with Acupuncture

Acupuncture has its roots in ancient Chinese medicine, but it has
become popular worldwide for the treatment of many ailments.
The basic theory underlying acupuncture is that there are channels of energy, or Qi, called *meridians*, which run throughout the
body. There are 360 acupuncture points on the meridians. When
a person is in a state of good health, energy flows freely along these
channels. In disease, the energy flow is disrupted, leading to symptoms. Acupuncture applied at specific points is thought to release
the energy and redirect its flow. In some cases, electrical stimuli are
used with the acupuncture needles to increase the effect; this is
called *electro-acupuncture*.

Two very small trials examining acupuncture for the treatment
of IBS have been performed with contradictory results. Despite the
lack of data, many people report having pursued acupuncture to
successfully treat abdominal pain, bloating, and nausea. Acupuncture is generally safe if it is performed by a licensed acupuncturist,
and it might be a good adjunct treatment for people who are sensitive or intolerant to oral interventions. In severe cases, many acu-
puncturists use acupuncture in conjunction with herbal therapy.

Acupressure is similar to acupuncture, but instead of inserting
needles at the selected points, the meridians are stimulated using
firm thumb pressure or fingertip massage. The best-known example
of acupressure is Shiatsu massage.

Healing with Aromatherapy

Aromatherapy involves massaging areas of the body, using a preparation of fragrant essential oils extracted from herbs, flowers, and fruits. Massage of the stomach and lower back can often be helpful in stimulating a constipated bowel, relieving gas and distension, or easing the pain associated with IBS. You can visit a qualified aromatherapist for a massage or you can do it yourself. You might also find it helpful to apply alternate hot and cold compresses to your abdomen to stimulate circulation. (See "Therapeutic Heat" below.)

THERAPEUTIC HEAT

Direct heat is a tremendously effective muscle relaxant, and it can be wonderfully beneficial for most IBS symptoms. If you have access to a Jacuzzi, steam bath, or sauna, take advantage of it and try engaging in regular sessions of heat-induced bliss. A hot-oil massage, especially with aromatherapy, can work wonders, too.

Make a particular effort to try heat therapy immediately before any upcoming stressful event. A simple hot bath will do, or even a long, hot shower. You can also wrap yourself up in an electric blanket, or apply a hot water bottle, hot pack, or heat wraps directly to your abdomen.

To make your own aromatherapy massage oil, you need carrier oil (a base oil used to dilute essential oils), such as grapeseed. Add ten to twenty drops of essential oil to one tablespoonful of the carrier oil. Rosemary, chamomile, and marjoram, used separately or blended with oil of black pepper and fennel, are often recommended for IBS. Other helpful essential oils are listed below:

♦ For constipation: black pepper, cardamom, fennel, ginger, lemon, peppermint, rosemary, and sandalwood

♦ For gas and bloating: cardamom, coriander, dill, and peppermint

♦ For diarrhea: basil, chamomile, lemon, orange, and peppermint

♦ For abdominal pain: chamomile, clove, eucalyptus, ginger, lavender, neroli, peppermint, rosemary, and thyme

Once your oils are blended, you are ready for your massage:

1. Place the container of diluted oil in a bowl of warm water to gently heat it.

2. Lie down in a warm, quiet room and expose your abdomen.

3. Place some warmed oil on your hands and gently massage your abdomen. Work clockwise; start by the right side of your groin and massage with slow, circular movements, pressing deeply without causing discomfort. Work your way up to your rib cage, across your abdomen, and down the left side of your groin again. Your massage should last at least five minutes. You might find it easier to get a partner or friend to do this for you.

Traditional Chinese Medicine (TCM)

TCM is based on a holistic approach. Thus, a complete and proper diagnosis involves an analysis of your whole body, not just your abdominal area. For instance, your practitioner might check your tongue to determine whether the coating on your tongue is related to your IBS systems. When you experience pain or discomfort—as with the symptoms of IBS—TCM practitioners believe that your body is out of balance.

TCM uses a variety of different natural treatment methods to correct an imbalance. Chinese herbal medicine is one such method. Specific herbs are prescribed to treat specific symptoms and aid the body in healing. For example, if you experience bloating, an herb that helps relieve bloating will be recommended.

Experienced TCM practitioners are well versed in the herbs that can be used for the treatment of IBS, but they will have to make sure the right ones for your individual case are recommended. *Note*: You will probably need to consume the herbal concoction a few times before you start to experience results. As in most natural treatments, TCM requires time for healing to take place.

Acupuncture (see above) is another natural IBS treatment that is part of TCM. There are also TCM exercises, such as t'ai chi, yoga (see below), and qigong, that you can do to promote relaxation and to quiet your mind. This helps to improve overall well-being. Some people believe that using TCM as a natural IBS treatment option is a good idea, and there have been a limited number of research studies that suggest it might have positive benefits. However, make sure you get proper referrals for a good TCM practitioner before seeking a consultation.

Healing with Homeopathy

Homeopathy operates on the principle that a specific substance, which in large doses will cause the symptoms of an illness, can be used in minute doses to relieve the same symptoms. Treatments are prescribed according to your symptoms rather than the disease, so two people with IBS, having differing symptoms, would be given different treatments. You can consult a private homeopathic practitioner or buy remedies direct from a pharmacy. Although it is best to consult a specialist, you might find the following remedies helpful for the specific symptoms listed. Your symptoms might initially get worse, but you need to persevere, because this is often a sign that the remedy is working:

- Constipation with no desire to empty the bowels: Alumina 6c
- Constipation with spasm and an urge to empty the bowels: Nux vomica 6c
- Diarrhea with nervousness and anxiety: Argentum 6c
- Diarrhea with flatulence and burning of the rectum: Aloe 6c
- Diarrhea and foul-smelling stools: Sulphur 6c or podophyllum
- Exhausting diarrhea and flatulence: China 6c

♦ Alternating diarrhea and constipation: Argentum 6c or lilium tigrinum

♦ Diarrhea with abdominal pain: Arsenicum album 6c

♦ Diarrhea brought on by drinking coffee: Psorinum 6c

♦ Cramping bowel pain: Colocynthis or Mag. Phos. 6c

♦ Bloating and distension: Lycopodium 6c

♦ IBS symptoms that are worse in the late afternoon and early evening: Lycopodium

♦ IBS and extreme fatigue: Mag. Phos

♦ An itching, burning rectum with oozing: Sulphur

Healing with Hypnotherapy

Hypnotherapy has been shown to be effective for the treatment of IBS in several clinical trials. For example, in a review of fourteen previous clinical studies published in the *American Journal of Clinical Hypnosis* in 2005 the conclusion was that hypnotherapy produces consistently significant results in IBS.

Hypnotherapy usually requires weekly individual sessions over several months, but it has also been tried in groups and with self-instruction. Hypnotherapy typically involves progressive relaxation followed by suggestions of soothing imagery and sensations focused on an individual's symptoms. Improvements in overall well-being, quality of life, abdominal pain, constipation, and bloating have been noted. A hypnotherapist will ask for some background details about your IBS experiences and symptoms. Then, the therapist will coax you into a state of extreme relaxation and take you through a program of suggestion. For example, you might be asked to imagine that when you hold your hand over your stomach, a healing warmth flows into your abdomen, or you might be asked to visualize a fully working digestive system. You will remain in complete control of your actions at all times. A therapist might record each session onto a CD or audiocassette, which will allow you to maintain the benefits of the therapy between sessions by allowing you to replay the tape whenever the need arises.

One of the difficulties with hypnosis is that it is very dependent on the therapist, and it might be difficult to find a therapist who is both trained in hypnosis and knowledgeable about functional GI disorders. Additionally, like many alternative therapies, it can be costly, and often it is not covered by insurance plans. If you are unable to attend regular sessions with a hypnotherapist or cannot afford the sessions, there are self-hypnosis programs and cassettes available that are designed to be used at home.

Movement Therapy

No studies on IBS are available for specific movement therapies, such as yoga or t'ai chi. It has been shown, however, that relaxation-response meditation aids the symptoms of abdominal pain, bloating, flatulence, and diarrhea, based on a small study. These types of therapies are particularly attractive, because they have no potential worrisome side effects, and they might be helpful for relieving symptoms outside the GI tract. They also promote general stress reduction.

Yoga—or, really, hatha yoga—is a set of practices that uses posture, breathing techniques, and relaxation to increase suppleness, calm the body and mind, and boost health and well-being. Like most therapies, it is best to learn from a qualified teacher, who will be able to help you achieve mental control and the right yoga positions for your body. Breathing plays a particularly important role in yoga, because the breath is thought to embody the life force, or *prana*. The following simple poses, which should be held for at least thirty seconds, are good examples of yoga positions that might benefit specific symptoms of IBS.

Constipation

There are two positions that can help with constipation. The first is to lie flat on your back with your legs flat on the ground, and then slowly bring both your knees up into your chest.

The second is the seated forward bend (see Figure 6.1), in which you sit down with your back straight and your legs extended forward, and gently lean forward as far as you can.

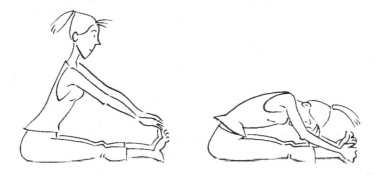

Figure 6.1 Seated forward bend

Diarrhea

Try the seated forward bend and the spinal twist (see Figure 6.2). For the spinal twist, lie flat on your back with your legs flat on the ground. Slowly bring one leg into the chest, and then twist it over the other leg so that it lies flat on the floor at your side.

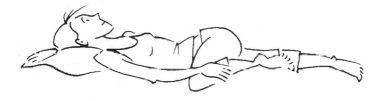

Figure 6.2 Spinal twist

Gas

Try lying flat on your back and then bringing both knees into your chest. You could also try the relieving posture (see Figure 6.3 on the next page), in which you bring one leg into your chest and gently push it into your body with your arms.

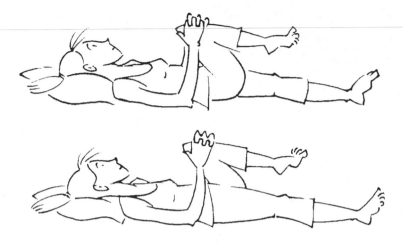

Figure 6.3 Relieving posture

Bloating

For bloating, if you are very fit and flexible (and not in too much discomfort), try a shoulder stand. Another effective method is the arch-and-release technique (see Figure 6.4), in which you "stand" on your hands and knees and arch your back like a cat.

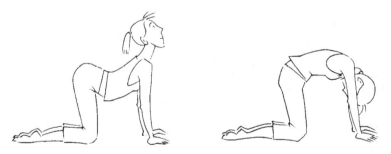

Figure 6.4: Arch and release (also known as cat and cow)

Indigestion

Try the cobra and backward bend (see Figures 6.5 and 6.6). For the cobra, lie flat on your stomach and gently arch up the upper part of your body, leaving your hips on the floor.

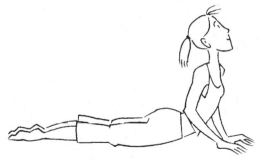

Figure 6.5 Cobra

For the backward bend, put your hands on the back of your waist and gently tilt your shoulders, neck, and head backward as far as you can go without losing your balance.

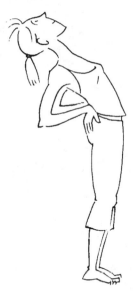

Figure 6.6 Backward bend

Reflexology

Reflexology is based on the theory that different "reflex" zones on the feet correspond to other areas of the body. So, if one part of the foot is suffering from tension, a corresponding part of the body is also suffering. The feet, therefore, form a map of the body that can be used to treat symptoms.

By treating the problems in the foot, the corresponding body part will also be healed. Therapists might also treat your hands in a similar way. Reflexologists often say that stress and tension can be relieved by reflexology, but they also claim success with many other conditions, including digestive problems. During a reflexology session the therapist will take a background history and ask you questions about your symptoms. The therapist will then treat you by applying pressure to various parts of your feet, and possibly your hands. This treatment should not be painful, although it might be uncomfortable when areas of particular tension are massaged. Although there are no studies to prove that reflexology can be of benefit to people with IBS, some people with the condition have found it helpful, because it can relieve fatigue and a number of stress-related symptoms, such as tension, digestive problems, and PMS.

If you are unable to visit a therapist, you and a partner or friend can easily learn how to give each other a foot massage by following the steps described below:

- ◆ Soak your feet in warm water for about ten minutes. You might wish to include drops of your favorite essential oil or bath salts. Peppermint or lavender oil is preferred by many. Make sure your feet are completely dry before starting the massage.

- ◆ Apply a moderate amount of cream or oil to your hands for comfort and ease. Make sure your hands are warm to avoid discomfort. Mineral oil is good because it is not absorbed into the skin and wipes off cleanly.

- ◆ Begin by stroking the top of the foot, moving in the direction from toe to ankle. Then continue by stroking the sole of the foot; first more gently, and then with increasing pressure.

- ◆ Make circular motions with your thumb and fingers over the sole of the foot, using more pressure in areas like the heel or ball of the foot. Start from the top and work your way down. Do not neglect the sides.

♦ Holding the foot with one hand, use the other hand to rotate the foot; first at the ankle, and then near the ball of the foot. Be gentle. Repeat about five times in each direction.

♦ Knead the sole by holding the foot with one hand and making a fist with the other, using moderate pressure to push the fist into the sole. Give attention to the arch.

♦ Beginning with the big toe and working toward the little toe, manipulate each toe individually. Roll the toe between your thumb and forefinger as you slide your fingers down the toe to the end, applying gentle pressure. Gently squeeze the end of each toe.

♦ Slide your index fingerbetween each toe about five times.

♦ To complete the massage, use your thumb and fingers to again make circular motions over the sole. End by stroking the sole and instep.

♦ Wipe off any excess cream or oil with a soft towel. Slip into thick socks to retain moisturizing, or slippers will suffice.

♦ Try to give equal attention to both feet because the body abhors asymmetry.

Chapter 7

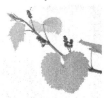

Healing IBS with Stress Management

Victoria, age 27

I feel my symptoms are connected with emotional problems and stress. Before I was diagnosed with IBS I used to think the symptoms were something I did to myself. I grew up with a father who verbally abused me. He would constantly shout at me when I was at the dinner table, and that's when my abdominal pains started. I was never good enough for him, and although I worked hard to impress him, it seemed the harder I worked the more he shouted. In my late teens I started to avoid eating at the dinner table, and eventually I didn't want to eat at all. Fortunately, around that same time my mother divorced my father and we moved away. I got some counseling and graduated from the university with honors. I'm much happier now, and I'm eating more or less normally again. My emotional problems are behind me, but I still find that when I'm under stress my IBS symptoms flare up.

Stress stimulates excessive adrenaline production, which goes on to upset the rhythmic muscle contractions of the gut. The stress response can also change the acid content of the stomach, killing the friendly bacteria that are needed for digestive harmony. Given that people with IBS are prone to suffering from irregular gut muscle contractions anyway, it's easy to see why stress can be such a powerful trigger or, in some cases, cause the onset of IBS. Several interesting studies have actually shown a direct link between emotional stressors and subsequent IBS flares.

Fortunately, it's easy for the body to reverse its response to stress. Your body begins to relax as soon as your brain cancels signals to the central nervous system, and within about three minutes the panic messages cease and relaxation begins. Your body can't tell whether the relaxation response was triggered by a change in circumstances or your attitude; either way, the symptoms are the same. So just as stress can make IBS symptoms worse, reversing stress and learning how to relax might help ease symptoms.

An important part of the IBS healing plan is to learn techniques for reducing anxiety and stress. The methods listed below can be helpful in promoting relaxation and minimizing stress-related IBS. Some can be learned in the time it takes to read this page, while others take a little more practice, but there's something here for everyone! With the exception of behavioral therapy, counseling, and Reiki, they are all techniques you can try on your own.

Techniques to Help Calm Your Mind and Your Colon

Breathing

Most of us, especially when we are nervous or stressed, breathe rapidly and shallowly from the chest, but some people find that when they learn how to breathe from the diaphragm instead, it helps to promote relaxation. Deep breathing is an easy stress reliever that has numerous benefits for the body, including oxygenating the blood, which "wakes up" the brain, relaxes the muscles, and quiets the mind. Breathing exercises are especially helpful because you can do them anywhere, and they work quickly so you can de-stress in a flash. The basic stress-relieving breathing exercise below is a great place to start.

Basic Stress-Relieving Breathing Exercise

- ◆ Sit or stand in a relaxed position.

- ◆ Slowly inhale through your nose, counting to five in your head.

- ◆ Let the air out of your mouth, counting to eight in your head as it leaves your lungs. Repeat several times. That's it!

Tips

- ◆ Let your abdomen expand outwards as you breathe, rather than raising your shoulders. This is a more relaxed and natural way to breathe, and it helps your lungs fill more deeply with fresh air and release more "old" air.

- ◆ You can perform this breathing exercise just a few times to release tension, or for several minutes as a form of meditation.

- ◆ If you like, you can make your throat a little tighter as you exhale so the air comes out like a whisper. This type of breathing is used in some forms of yoga, and it can add additional tension relief.

Behavioral Therapy

One approach to coping with IBS is behavioral therapy. This is because stress and anxiety can worsen IBS symptoms, and behavioral therapy can help you cope with these feelings, thus reducing some IBS symptoms. It's not known what about pressure and worry triggers stomach pain, discomfort, diarrhea, or constipation, but learning how to manage emotional reactions effectively seems to prevent or ease suffering. Behavioral therapy helps people learn how to cope better with pain and discomfort, and how to relieve stressful situations in order to ward off severe IBS symptoms.

Unfortunately, behavioral therapy is not a cure-all. Some studies have shown the strategy does help to ease stress-related symptoms of IBS, but others show it does nothing for the symptoms of constipation and constant stomachaches. Other studies show that it is best used with standard medical care. Before starting any form of therapy, talk with your doctor about how it might fit into your overall treatment plan. There are many different types of behavioral therapy. The following techniques have worked for some people with IBS.

Relaxation Therapy

The goal of relaxation therapy is to get the mind and body into a calm, peaceful state. Techniques include meditation, progressive muscle relaxation (tensing and loosening individual muscles), deep breathing, and guided imagery (visualization).

Biofeedback

This strategy uses an electrical device to help people recognize their body's response to stress. Participants are taught, with the machine's help, to slow down their heart rate to create a more relaxed state. After a few sessions, people are able to calm themselves down on their own.

Hypnotherapy

Participants enter an altered state of consciousness, either with the assistance of a trained professional or on their own (after training). In this altered condition, verbal suggestions are made to help them imagine their pain going away. (See section earlier in this chapter.)

Cognitive Behavioral Therapy

This is a form of psychotherapy that teaches you to analyze negative, distorted thoughts and replace them with more positive, realistic thoughts.

Traditional Psychotherapy

In traditional psychotherapy, a trained mental-health professional helps people work out their conflicts and learn to understand their feelings.

Counseling

Working with a counselor to figure out how to cope with stress and IBS is one approach to living a more relaxed life. A study conducted through the Department of Medicine at Humboldt University in Berlin, and published in the May 2002 in the *American Journal of Gastroenterology*, showed that when a group of people with IBS attended ten sessions of behavioral therapy lasting one hour each over a ten-week period, they felt more in control of their health and agreed that they had a better quality of life than those who did not partake in therapy. During the therapy sessions, participants were provided with information about IBS, an analysis of their own unique symptoms, and training in coping strategies and problem-solving. If counseling isn't an option, talking with loved ones or friends or linking up with others with IBS via a support group or website are other ways to ease stress.

Exercise

Whether you have IBS or not, exercise is as important as a good diet for staying healthy both physically and emotionally. But are you doing it regularly? If you aren't, here are some very good reasons why you should.

Exercise firms your abdominal muscles and triggers the intestinal contractions that keep your digestive system moving smoothly, which in turn helps with the passage of gas, reduces bloating and cramping, and results in more regular bowel movements. Exercise is also one of the best stress relievers.

Research shows that regular exercise can help relieve IBS symptoms, but you don't have to run a marathon to enjoy the benefits. As little as thirty minutes a day of light physical activity helps—for example, housework, walking the dog, climbing the stairs, or mowing the lawn. Plus, you don't have to do all thirty minutes of activity at once.

Although at least thirty minutes of activity a day needs to be part of your IBS healing plan, to fully enjoy all the benefits of exercise—including lowered blood pressure and lowered cholesterol levels, weight loss, and a reduction of anxiety and stress—you do have to work a bit harder and must plan and follow through with a well-rounded exercise program. Research shows that people with IBS are less likely to exercise than people without it, so if you haven't been exercising regularly, then get started. The simple exercise tips described below will show you that this isn't as exhausting or as complicated as it sounds.

GETTING STARTED WITH EXERCISE

Most people can begin gradual, moderate exercise on their own. If you think there is a reason that you might not be able to exercise safely, talk to your doctor before beginning a new exercise program. In particular, your doctor needs to know if you have heart trouble, high blood pressure, or arthritis, or if you often feel dizzy or have chest pains.

Simple ways to increase your activity levels during the day include, for example, standing rather than sitting, getting off the bus a few stops early, and taking the stairs instead of the elevator.

Start your more formal program by exercising three or more times a week for five to fifteen minutes until you have gradually and slowly worked up to at least thirty minutes, four to six times a week. Getting to thirty minutes five times a week might take several weeks or even a few months to achieve, so don't worry if you feel exhausted after your first 10-minute session. Just stick with it, and you'll soon find that your fitness levels and enjoyment have increased. If you don't think you can find a spare thirty minutes, try to include several short bouts of activity in a day, say three slots of ten minutes each. Exercising during a lunch-break or on your way to do errands might help you add physical activity to a busy schedule.

Choose an activity that you enjoy, can start slowly, and can increase gradually as you become used to it. Walking is very popular and does not require special equipment. Other good ways to exercise include swimming, biking, and gentle trampoline use. Exercise is any physical activity that raises the heart rate. You don't necessarily have to join a gym.

(cont'd.)

> Start with an activity you can do comfortably. As a rule of thumb, when you are exercising you should be slightly out of breath but not so out of breath that you can't hold a conversation with someone else. Stop if you find yourself panting or huffing and puffing. These signs mean you're exercising too hard.

Sample Gentle Exercise Plan
for Walking, Swimming, Cycling, and Jogging

You should start your exercise session with a gradual warm-up period. During this time period (about five to ten minutes), you should slowly stretch your muscles first, and then gradually increase your level of activity. For example, begin walking slowly and then pick up the pace. After you have finished exercising, cool down for about five to ten minutes. Again, stretch your muscles and let your heart rate slow down gradually. You can use the same stretches as in the warm-up period.

Walking

Walking is great. No expertise or equipment is required; you can do it anytime and it's free! What's more, provided you do it regularly and for long enough periods of time, walking can be just as beneficial as more vigorous activities like jogging.

How to Start a Walking Program

♦ Take a 10-minute walk, twice a day.

♦ Walk every day.

♦ Gradually extend your pace.

♦ Walk for longer periods of time or for farther distances.

♦ Walk and swing your arms at the same time.

♦ Walk up one or two gentle slopes.

♦ Walk up steeper slopes.

Aim to walk briskly (swinging your arms) for thirty to forty-five minutes each day. This should include at least one reasonably steep slope. (*Please note:* This might take you several months to achieve, so don't be in a hurry.) Remember, exercise is for LIFE!

Swimming

For most people, especially those who are very overweight, swimming is even better than walking.

How to start and then extend yourself. As with walking, you should start by going to the pool twice a week for a gentle 15-minute swim. Gradually increase the length of your swim and your work rate while in the water. Aim to build up to about thirty minutes a day, or forty-five minutes twice a week.

Cycling/Cycle-Machine, Trampoline, or Jogging

Your aim with these activities is the same as for walking or swimming. Start with a short easy routine of ten to fifteen minutes per day and gradually work up to about thirty minutes a day. Gradually increase the activity without straining yourself. If you choose jogging, please invest in a good pair of running shoes that offer cushioned support; if you're a woman, invest in a good sports bra for use with all activities.

If you haven't exercised for a while, it's really important to find a form of exercise you enjoy and to start slowly and build gradually. If you attempt "too much, too soon," it will lead to soreness, fatigue, and/or injuries. Work at your own level, start out slowly, and gradually increase the duration and level of difficulty as your body progresses.

In addition to your regular workouts, don't forget to do some gentle toning exercises, such as push-ups, sits-ups, lunges, and so on. Do your toning exercises for about twenty minutes three to four times a week. If you don't like going to the gym for a class, there are plenty of fitness videos, books, and magazines that can give you advice on how to perform toning exercises correctly. Simple things like carrying your grocery items instead of using a cart or walking up the stairs can also help you tone your muscles. You could also try the exercises below, which stretch and tone the muscles, and also help relieve IBS symptoms. (See also the yoga exercises in the previous chapter.)

Exercises

Abdominal training. Sit on the floor with your knees slightly bent and your back straight. You can hold your arms straight out in front of you for balance, or you can cross them over your chest. From this sitting position, slowly lower your back toward the floor until your shoulders are just a few inches above the floor. Pause, and then slowly roll back up to a sitting position. As you do this exercise, always press the small of your back downwards, rather than arching your back, in order to prevent strain. Repeat ten times.

Stomach contractions. Stand up with your hands on your knees. Inhale and exhale fully. With your breath held out, pull your stomach in as far as you can and then release it all the way out. Repeat this contraction five times in one exhalation.

Abdominal windmills. Lie on your back and bring your knees up to your chest. Then move both knees to your right, touching the floor on your right side. Then, keeping your knees together, revolve to the left, touching the floor on your left side. Hold your knees with your hands if you need to. Repeat ten times.

◆ ◆ ◆

Getting fit, like healthy eating, is not an overnight proposition; it's a lifestyle commitment. Sadly, only one-third of the people who begin an exercise program are typically still exercising by the end of their first year. The good news is that with some strategizing and planning, you can beat the drop-out odds and make a successful transition to a lifestyle that incorporates exercise. Here are some tips to help you stay motivated:

♦ *Find a fitness partner.* Studies show that sticking with exercise is generally more likely if the family or a friend is included in the commitment to exercise. Find a walking partner, play tennis with your spouse, or go rollerblading with the children.

♦ *Start an exercise log or journal.* An exercise log or journal is an excellent way to chart your progress and provide motivation. Nothing beats the feeling of success as you read through your accomplishments. Exercise logs can take on many forms: a calendar to record your workouts, a daily journal to record your feelings and goals, a computerized exercise log, or a log purchased at a bookstore. The key is to select a log or journal that fits your needs and provides you with the kind of information that is meaningful to you.

♦ *Schedule your workouts.* Exercise must be a priority in order to establish it as a lifestyle practice. Make time for your workouts and schedule them on your daily calendar or planner.

♦ *Dress the part.* Wear comfortable clothes that are appropriate for exercising; they will help you feel more like working out. If you exercise at a gym, put your exercise clothes in a bag and set it beside the door the night before. Then all you have to do is grab your bag on the way out the next day.

♦ *Entertain yourself.* If you exercise alone, consider using a portable music device to listen to your favorite music or books on cassette and help keep you entertained during your workout. Many pieces of exercise equipment have racks that fit on to the console to hold reading material. If you exercise at home, turn on some music or place the television within viewing range.

♦ *Make exercise non-negotiable.* Think of exercise as something you do without question, like brushing your teeth or going to work. Taking the lifestyle perspective will help you make exercise a habit.

Massage

There are many types of massage, and all of them are thought to help improve circulation, calm muscle pain and spasm, and relieve stress. Some people with IBS find therapeutic abdominal massage to be extremely helpful.

THERAPEUTIC ABDOMINAL MASSAGE FOR IBS

- Put a tablespoonful of massage oil on a warmer for ten minutes (e.g., on top of a radiator). Suitable massage oils are almond oil or grapeseed oil.
- Add one or two (no more) drops of one of the essential oils listed below.
- Lie down in a comfortable position and gently massage the oil into your abdomen using slow circular movements in a clockwise direction (i.e., up your right side, across your tummy button, and down your left side).
- Play some gentle music and relax while you massage. Nicer still, get your spouse or a friend to perform this massage process on you; this can be very soothing!
- Oils for constipation: marjoram, rosemary, fennel.
- Oils for diarrhea:chamomile, lavender, neroli.

Note: Never use these oils full strength; always dilute them in a massage/carrier oil (see above section on aromatherapy).

Meditation

Research has shown that meditation can help relax the body, and many people with stress-related IBS find that it helps. There are numerous books, CDs, and classes that can teach you how to meditate, but even without using formal meditation techniques it can help to take some time out of your day to sit or lie down and simply stop doing anything. To experiment with meditation on your own, find a quiet place where you won't be interrupted. Sit in a firm chair with your back straight and try one of the following forms of meditation, each of which has a different focus object.

Mantra Meditation

For this meditation, choose a word like "peace" or a neutral sound like "ahhh" and then repeat that word or sound each time you breathe out.

Gazing Meditation

Look at an object, perhaps a flower or photograph, to focus your attention. Keeping your eyes relaxed, gaze, rather than stare, at the object. Don't think about the object, just look at it.

Breathing Meditation

This involves focusing on the rise and fall of your breath. Take a deep breath, focus on the inhalation, pause before you exhale, and then exhale and pause before you inhale again. Try to clear your mind of all thoughts except your breathing processes.

Walking Meditation

As you walk, focus your attention on each foot as it contacts the ground. When your mind wanders away from your feet or legs or the feeling of your body walking, refocus your attention. To deepen your concentration, don't look around, but rather keep your gaze in front of you.

Before each meditation session, inhale deeply, and then exhale to release any tension. During your meditation, if thoughts about your daily life creep into your mind (which they will do), accept them and let them drift away. Try meditation for five minutes a day and then work up to fifteen minutes a day; the more you practice, the better your experience will be, and, hopefully, the more relaxed and calm you will become.

Music Therapy

Music is one of the most commonly used methods for stress reduction. Certain types of music definitely help relieve stress. Many studies have been done on the role of music in relieving stress, and it has been determined that it is the rhythm or beat that relieves stress. While listening to music there is an increase in the depth of breathing, which provides more oxygen and therefore more energy to the body. Also, music causes the brain to secrete serotonin, which acts as a mood stabilizer. So what are you waiting for? Turn on some soothing classical or modern music, put your feet up, and relax.

Reiki

This Japanese art of healing is based on a philosophy that the laying on of hands on different parts of the body can balance the mind, body, and spirit by releasing blocked energy and helping the body heal itself. Although no studies have shown Reiki to be specifically of benefit to people with IBS, it's gentle and relaxing, and some people say it works wonders.

Relaxation

When performed correctly, relaxation exercises can lead to a profound feeling of calm. Simple ways to relax include sitting quietly and reading a book or a magazine for an hour, using an aromatherapy candle to fill the air with a relaxing aroma, chatting with friends, or enjoying a candlelit warm bath, scented with a few drops of relaxing aromatherapy oil.

For a deep relaxation exercise like the one in the box below— which tenses and relaxes different muscle groups—you will need to set aside half an hour, preferably after a long soak in a warm bath.

DEEP RELAXATION EXERCISE

Sit in a comfortable chair—reclining armchairs are ideal. A bed is okay, too. Get as comfortable as possible—no tight clothes, no shoes, and don't cross your legs. Take a deep breath; let it out slowly. Repeat this. What you will be doing in this exercise is alternately tensing and relaxing specific groups of muscles. After tensing, a muscle will become more relaxed than prior to the tensing. Concentrate on the feel of the muscles, specifically the contrast between tension and relaxation. In time you will recognize tension in any specific muscle and be able to reduce that tension.

(cont'd.)

Don't tense muscles other than those in the specific group involved at each step. Don't hold your breath, grit your teeth, or squint! Breathe slowly and evenly, and think only about the tension-relaxation contrast. Note that each step is really two steps—one cycle of tension-relaxation for each set of opposing muscles.

Do the entire sequence once a day if you can, until you feel you are able to control your muscle tension. Be careful: If you have problems with pulled muscles, broken bones, or any other medical contraindication for physical activities, consult your doctor before you attempt these relaxation exercises.

1. *Hands.* The fists are tensed, then relaxed. The fingers are extended, then relaxed.

2. *Biceps and triceps.* The biceps are tensed (make a muscle—but shake your hands to ensure you are not tensing them into a fist), then relaxed (drop your arms down into the chair—really drop them). Next, the triceps are tensed (try to bend your arms the wrong way), then relaxed (drop them).

3. *Shoulders.* Pull them back (careful with this one), then relax them. Push the shoulders forward (hunch), then relax.

4. *Neck (lateral).* With the shoulders straight and relaxed, turn your head slowly to the right, as far as you can; then relax. Next, turn your head to the left; then relax.

5. *Neck (forward).* Dig your chin into your chest, then relax (straining the head back is not recommended as you could strain your neck).

6. *Mouth.* Open your mouth as far as possible, then relax. Next, bring the lips together (purse) as tightly as possible; then relax them.

7. *Tongue (extended and retracted).* With your mouth open, extend the tongue as far as possible; then relax (let it sit in the bottom of your mouth). Next, move it back in your throat as far as possible; then relax.

8. *Tongue (roof and floor).* Dig your tongue into the roof of your mouth; then relax. Dig it into the bottom of your mouth; then relax.

9. *Eyes.* Open them as wide as possible (furrow your brow); relax. Close your eyes tightly (squint); then relax. Make sure you

(cont'd.)

completely relax the eyes, forehead, and nose after each of the tensings—this can actually be quite difficult.

10. *Breathing.* Take as deep a breath as possible—and then take in a little more; let it out and breathe normally for fifteen seconds. Let all of the air out of your lungs—and then a little more; inhale and breathe normally for fifteen seconds.

11. *Back.* With your shoulders resting on the back of the chair, push your body forward so that your back is arched; then relax. Be very careful with this one, or don't do it at all.

12. *Buttocks.* While sitting in a chair, tense the buttocks tightly and raise your pelvis slightly off the chair; then relax. Dig your buttocks into the chair; then relax.

13. *Thighs.* While sitting in a chair, extend your legs and raise them about six feet off the floor or the foot rest—but don't tense the stomach; then relax by gently dropping your legs. Dig your feet (heels) into the floor or foot rest; then relax.

14. *Stomach.* Pull in your stomach as far as possible; then relax completely. Push out your stomach or tense it as if you were preparing for a punch in the stomach; then relax.

15. *Calves and feet.* While sitting in a chair, point the toes (without raising the legs); then relax. Point the feet up as far as possible (beware of cramping; if you get a cramp or feel one coming on, shake your feet loose); then relax.

16. *Toes.* With legs relaxed, dig your toes into the floor; then relax. Bend the toes up as far as possible; then relax.

Finally, just relax for a while. As your practice progresses, you might wish to skip the steps that do not appear to be helpful to you. Then, after you've become an expert on your tension areas (after a few weeks), you can concern yourself only with these areas. Relaxation exercises such as these will not eliminate tension, but when tension arises you will know it immediately and be able to "tense-relax" it away, or even simply wish it away.

Visualization

You can reduce stress by merely using your imagination. Through visualization, which basically involves putting your imagination to work, you can ease stress by simply changing your thoughts. This technique builds on the idea that we are what we think; for example, if we think sad thoughts, we become sad, and if we think positive thoughts, we become more positive.

The following describes a simple visualization exercise that will enable you to relax deeply. It takes about ten or fifteen minutes. But once you've practiced it a few times, you can call on it instantly whenever you're in a stressful situation, before things get out of control.

VISUALIZATION EXERCISE

Sit in a chair. If it's comfortable for you to do so, keep your back straight. Breathe in through your nose to a count of four. Breathe out through your mouth to a count of eight. If you have some privacy, say "huh, huh, huh" at the end of the exhalation. Repeat the breaths four times.

Close your eyes. Tighten the muscles in your feet and then relax. Concentrate on feeling the muscles relax. Repeat. Tighten the muscles in your calves, relax, feel the relaxation, and repeat. Do the same with the muscles in your thighs, then with your buttocks, stomach, and lower back, then with your chest, then your upper back, then your shoulders, then arms, then hands, and then neck. Make a face, scrunching up your facial muscles, relax, and then repeat.

Think of a peaceful setting. It can be a beach or a forest or anything you choose. The important thing is that it's a place you've been where you felt relaxed and happy, and where you have had an all-around "good feeling."

Remember what the place looked like. Picture the details in your mind. Then remember the sounds you heard. Next, add in the smells you experienced. Then consider your sense of touch— what do you feel on your skin? Finally, add any taste elements that might pertain. Let all your senses work as you re-experience this place where you felt great.

Stay in this place in your mind for about five minutes, experiencing it as vividly as you can using all of your senses.

When you feel ready to do so, open your eyes. Stand up, lift your arms over your head, and stretch. Then drop your arms and shake them out.

At this point, think about the fact that you now know how to relax. It's a skill—a learned skill—and it is now included in your repertoire of coping behaviors. The more you practice these exercises, the more skillful you will become. Try one of these relaxation methods the next time you're feeling angry, frustrated, or upset. First, be aware of what's going on with your body. Do you feel any muscle tension? If so, where? Is your breathing different from the way it usually is? Is your heart beating faster? Do you feel any other changes in your body? Recognize the physical symptoms that signal you're under stress.

Stress is the body's natural response to danger. It floods the body with chemicals that prepare the body for "fight-or-flight." This was very helpful in ancient times when danger might be something like a wild animal that you needed to fight or run away from. But nowadays, many of the dangers that create stress are attacks not on our physical bodies, but on our sense of self-esteem. Neither fighting nor running are helpful in dealing with these situations, but the body continues to create fight-or-flight chemicals that interfere with your ability to cope. They can build up to such a great degree that they flood your system and keep you from thinking rationally.

When you realize that you are under stress, take a few deep breaths and recall the peaceful place that you experienced in the visualization exercise. Picture it again, vividly, in your mind. This will help your body cut down on the flow of stress chemicals before you become so flooded with them that you can't think straight.

Stress-Busters You Can Use Anytime, Anywhere

The following techniques can help when stress threatens to trigger your symptoms and you don't have time (or it isn't appropriate) to meditate, visualize for half an hour, or go for a run.

Fill Out Your Personal Space

Shrinking away from other people creates tension, so consciously relax your body, starting with the shoulders, and let yourself settle into your feet or your seat as if there were no one else around. Close your eyes or keep them slightly unfocused and turned downward. Now imagine that you are expanding into the space just surrounding your body, flowing into it with every exhaling breath, taking more space for yourself.

Try the Herbal Remedy Valerian

Valerian is a useful herb for stress-related anxiety and insomnia. This sedative has been shown to help people fall asleep faster and to sleep better and longer without causing a subsequent loss of concentration. Try drinking some kombucha tea, which contains stress-busting B vitamins and other micronutrients. Kombucha is made from a bacteria/yeast culture.

Daydream

For five minutes every hour, try to "shut down" and think of nothing but your perfect situation. This could be a dream holiday, ideal partner, or simply thinking about doing nothing at all. You will be surprised at how effectively this can lower stress levels. Daydreaming is a natural stress-busting technique. Allow your mind to wander for five minutes if you feel tense—maybe visualizing your favorite picture or happy memory to help you drift off.

Another type of visualization involves replacing an image you associate with tension with an image for relaxation. For example, you might visualize tension as a taut rope, the sound of thunder, the color red, pitch darkness, persistent hammering, or blinding white light. These images of tension can be made to soften and fade into images of relaxation. For instance, the taut rope loosens, the thunder subsides and is replaced by a light rain, red turns to light pink, the darkness begins to lighten, the pounding hammer is replaced by the murmur of cicadas and crickets, and the blinding white light softens to a sunset.

Ayurvedic Technique

Ayurvedic medicine originated in the Indus Valley some 5,000 years ago. It involves a number of herbal remedies, diet and lifestyle changes, and relaxing exercises designed to bring a troubled body or spirit back into harmony with the environment. Try this ayurvedic technique for soothing the brain: For as long as possible, gently massage the point above your nose in the middle of the forehead in a very light circular movement.

Aromatherapy

Certain aromas are thought to activate the production of the brain's feel-good chemical, serotonin. Place a few drops of the following aromatherapy oils on to a tissue to sniff when you feel stress levels rising: jasmine, neroli, lavender, chamomile, ylang ylang, vetiver, or clary sage. You might also want to use essential oils in your bath to help you unwind. When you feel tense, try one of the following: three drops of patchouli and three drops of sandalwood, three drops of rosewood and three drops of clary sage, or two drops of vetiver and jasmine. Or you might like to try two drops of peppermint or lemon essential oil on a tissue to inhale when stressed. If you prefer, you can also burn these oils in a vaporizer to help clarify and invigorate your mind and body.

De-clutter

Mess creates confusion and a sense of loss of power. If your desk/home/car is messy and disorganized, clean it up. You'll instantly feel more in control.

Release the Tension

Do you hunch your shoulders when you are stressed? Do you tighten your fists? Do you cross your arms? Do you wrap one leg around the other? Become aware of the way your body reacts when you are under stress. Then, when you feel yourself going into a stress position, do the opposite—release your shoulders, stretch out your hands, uncross your arms or legs, and don't forget to breathe. Stop frowning and relax your jaw by gently resting the tip of your tongue for a second behind your top front teeth. At the same time, try to consciously relax your facial muscles and let your shoulders drop down and away from your ears by an inch or two—you'll be amazed to find how much tension you were holding in your body.

Chamomile

One of the best herbs for relieving tension is chamomile because it has a gentle sedative effect. Drink a cup anytime you feel tense to help you to relax. If you drink a cup of chamomile tea before you go to bed, it will help you get to sleep.

Stroke Your Pet

If you have a pet, stroke it. It's been proven to lower blood pressure and stress levels. If you haven't got a pet, why not give someone you love a hug—it will have the same effect.

Write It Down

When it all seems too much, grab a pen and paper and write down what you are thinking about or what you need to do. Listing things on paper will also help you focus your mind and think clearly about what your priorities are, what can wait, and what can be delegated to someone else. Once a job has been dealt with, be sure to cross it off the list. It's satisfying and stress-busting to watch your list shrink!

Get Your Z's

Finally, one stress factor that can have a significant impact on IBS symptoms is sleep loss. Since a poor night's sleep results in fatigue and a corresponding lower stress-tolerance level, being tired allows IBS to be more easily triggered. A significant correlation has been noted between morning IBS symptoms and the quality of the previous night's sleep. In fact, morning IBS symptoms seem to rise or fall in direct association with the quality of the prior night's sleep. A less strong but still significant relationship was found between end-of-day IBS symptoms and the quality of sleep during the previous evening. Ensuring an adequate night's sleep should be a top priority for reducing stress-induced IBS symptoms.

So what is considered a good night's sleep? A good night's sleep boosts health and well-being, but research suggests that people who sleep for less than six hours tend to become irritable. Seven to eight hours seems to be the most beneficial, but six hours of good-quality sleep is far better than a restless eight.

Everyone has different sleep needs, but if one or more of the items on the list below apply to you, you are not getting enough good-quality sleep:

- You find waking up difficult.

- You yawn frequently.

- You fall asleep during the day.

- You lack energy.

- You feel drained or tired.

- You need caffeine and stimulants to get you through the day.

- You get dark circles under your eyes.

- You find it hard to concentrate.

- You become irritable for no apparent reason.

In addition to eating a healthy diet, there are many things you can do to improve your chances of obtaining a good night's sleep; for example:

- *Keep regular hours.* Going to bed and getting up at roughly the same time every day will train your body to sleep better by getting it into a regular rhythm.

- *Keep a pen and paper by your bedside.* Use these before lights-out to make a list of things that you need to tackle the next day, thus allowing you to "dump" worries that might prevent you from sleeping during the night.

♦ *Get some fresh air and sunlight.* Studies show that people who get their fair share of natural daylight tend to sleep better at night.

♦ *Take regular, moderate exercise.* Yoga, t'ai chi, or simply going for a brisk walk or swim are all ideal. But note that taking vigorous exercise too close to bedtime can hinder rather than help to provide quality sleep.

♦ *Make sure your bedroom is not too hot, cold, noisy, or light.* An overheated, underventilated bedroom can cause you to awaken in the middle of the night. Likewise, try to make your bedroom as quiet and dark as possible. A comfortable bed—not too hard, soft, or small—and a high-quality pillow can also help create a good sleeping environment.

♦ *Avoid excess alcohol.* A small nightcap might help you to wind down and get to sleep, but alcohol is likely to interrupt your sleep later in the night.

♦ *Avoid coffee and tea—especially in the evening.* Both are stimulants, which can interfere with falling asleep and prevent deep sleep. Even the caffeine in sodas can affect the quality of sleep. Research also shows that caffeine can have an effect on some people if taken earlier in the day, so it might be worth looking at your overall intake, including what you consume in the morning and afternoon.

♦ *Avoid overindulging late at night.* Doing this can ruin your sleep patterns.

♦ *Don't smoke.* Yes, it's bad for sleep, too. Nicotine is a stimulant, and smokers take longer to fall asleep, awaken more often, and experience more sleep disruption.

♦ *Drink a cup of herbal tea.* Unlike black or green tea, which contain caffeine, most herbal teas will relax rather than stimulate you.

♦ *Eat bananas and avocados.* Both are good sources of vitamin B, which can help with sleep problems caused by adrenal stress. You can also buy a good vitamin B complex—or astragalus, the herb favoured by Chinese healers—and take it at bedtime.

♦ *Sprinkle a few drops of lavender oil on your pillow.* This is a natural soother.

♦ *Make love.* Sex is nature's best soporific. Even if it doesn't send you to sleep, it's a lot more fun than staying awake, and it's also a fantastic tension reliever.

♦ *Try to relax before going to bed.* A warm bath—especially on cold, winter nights—will gently warm and relax you. Yoga, deep breathing, or listening to soothing music can also help relax the mind and body. Some people like listening to CDs of whale or water sounds. Your doctor (or local music store employee) might be able to suggest a helpful relaxation CD.

♦ *Use "trigger pictures" to help you relax.* Try to conjure mental images of a favorite or fantasy place or moment—for example, a great birthday party or an idyllic holiday spot—as a way of triggering feelings of relaxation and well-being.

♦ *Play mind games.* Counting sheep is the most famous technique, but there are countless others; for example, consider the following:
  – Imagine a room covered wall-to-wall and floor-to-ceiling with black velvet.
  – Describe your home village, town, or city in the greatest possible detail, as though to a complete stranger.
  – Keep repeating the words "Sleep, Sleep, Sleep, Sleep" very slowly until you drop off.
  – Numb the brain by making it perform a dull, boring task, such as repeating the words "Um" and "Ah" in ever increasing numbers. The "Ums" must always be two more than the "Ahs," giving the following sequence:

    a. Um
    b. Um Um Ah
    c. Um Um Um Um Ah Ah … and so on.

♦ *Don't just lie there; do something.* If you really can't sleep, don't just lie there fretting about it. Get up and do something you find relaxing—reading, watching television, or whatever—until you feel sleepy again. When you start to feel tired, go back to bed.

Chapter 8

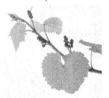

Working with Your Doctor

Luke, age 31

There's only one thing that relieves my diarrhea, and that is Lomotil. I have to go to my doctor every few months for a fix, but it works. I don't like being so dependent on it, but I'd rather use it than live my life running to the bathroom every half hour. I hope I'll find another way someday, but my doctor thinks it's okay for me now.

Charlotte, age 61

For about ten years I've had problems with constipation. I feel too young to have this problem, and I was certainly too young when I got it. Doctors have constantly told me to include more fiber in my diet, but it hasn't helped, and last year my doctor told me to take an antidepressant. I told him the reason I felt down was because I couldn't go to the bathroom like everyone else. He said antidepressant drugs might help, but they haven't. I've put on loads of weight and feel tired and thirsty all the time (typical symptoms of diabetes, although I'm told I don't have this). I don't feel like having sex at all. I thought being constipated was tough, but the additional problems are much worse.

In many ways having IBS forces you to become your own doctor, because it is up to you to take charge of your symptoms and find ways of dealing with them by watching your diet, exercising more, and managing your stress levels. However, this isn't to say you don't need your doctor's advice. Far from it! Your doctor is the person you need to turn to for advice about managing your symptoms and monitoring any changes that might need further testing. Teamwork between you and your doctor is essential, and a good relationship with your doctor provides an environment of understanding and concern that can make a huge difference.

Unfortunately, few doctors have specific training in how to manage IBS naturally through diet and lifestyle changes. Some might offer basic dietary advice, but for specific nutritional strategies and stress-management techniques you'll need to read this book. Even so, your doctor is the person you should contact to monitor your symptoms and check your progress—especially if your symptoms change or you experience warning signs not associated with IBS, such as blood in your stools.

If your doctor mentions drugs as a possible treatment option, bear in mind that although drugs might be able to offer you short-term relief, they are rarely effective in the long term. This is because drugs treat the symptoms of IBS rather than the cause of the digestive system irritation. In some cases traditional treatments might actually make IBS worse. For example, drugs like Tagamet inhibit the release of hydrochloric acid in the stomach, but the change in stomach acid alters the microbial environment throughout the digestive tract, which might actually exacerbate the digestive problems that caused the problems in the first place. Also, drugs often have unwanted side effects.

While the conventional approach to treating IBS has its downside, there might be times in your life when you need to resort to prescription medicine. Listed below is a rundown of the most commonly prescribed drugs and what symptoms they are meant to treat, plus possible side-effects and concerns about them.

Over-the-Counter Medications for IBS

Many people with IBS and their doctors turn to over-the-counter antidiarrhea drugs, such as Imodium, Maalox, and Kaopectate, for relief of IBS with diarrhea. In a 2002 comprehensive report by the American College of Gastroenterology, researchers found these drugs to be effective in controlling diarrhea. However, they did not help with other IBS symptoms, such as stomachache or swelling. Side effects of these drug treatments include discomfort, stomach cramping, and bloating, along with dry mouth, dizziness, and constipation. If you take an antidiarrhea drug, use the lowest dose possible and don't take it for an extended period of time.

Other over-the-counter products, such as Pepto-Bismol, antacids, and medicines for gas relief, are considered safe. Pepcid, Zantac, and Tagamet, which are taken for acid indigestion, are known as *H2 receptor antagonists*, and their job is to prevent histamines from releasing certain chemicals into your stomach. By blocking this activity, stomach acid and acid indigestion is reduced. The problem is that stomach acids don't cause IBS, so popping these pills won't help in the long term.

Bulk-forming laxatives, such as Citrucel, Konsyl, Metamucil, and Serutan, work by absorbing liquid in the intestines to help form a bulky stool that is soft enough to pass. These laxatives are generally considered a safe treatment for constipation, but they can interfere with the absorption of some medicines. They can also stimulate some degree of gas and bloating in the intestines.

Prescription Medicines

Many of the following medications can only be prescribed by doctors, although some (e.g., Imodium) can also be bought over-the-counter.

Antidepressants

Doctors might prescribe antidepressants for the abdominal pain associated with IBS. This does not necessarily mean that you are depressed. Low doses of antidepressants are known to block signals of pain to the brain. For people with IBS diarrhea, doctors will likely recommend a low dose of a type of antidepressant called *tricyclic antidepressants*, such as Pamelor, Elavil, and Tofranil. These drugs don't cause diarrhea like some of the newer antidepressants, such as Celexa, Seroxate, and Prozac. Common side effects of these antidepressants include dry mouth, blurred vision, and problems with constipation.

It's important to note that the dosage of antidepressants used for IBS is typically far lower than when the same drug is used for depression. It is also crucial that the doctor prescribing the drug is very familiar with its use for IBS, because different classes of antidepressants have varying side effects. Some can greatly worsen the diarrhea, constipation, and the pain of IBS, depending on the individual. In particular, SSRI antidepressants (for example, Prozac, Celexa, Zoloft, and Seroxate) stimulate serotonin production and can trigger severe IBS attacks in diarrhea-predominant individuals, although they might be helpful for constipation.

Conversely, tricyclic antidepressants (for example, Elavil) have the best track record of success for reducing diarrhea-predominant IBS symptoms, but people with constipation are not usually treated with these drugs because of the possibility of making the diarrhea worse. The long-term consequences of taking low-dose antidepressants for IBS are unknown, and this type of treatment should be discussed with your doctor.

Antispasmodics

Muscle spasms and gas in the gut cause much of the pain in IBS, and in some cases antispasmodics, like Donnatal, Levsin, Levbid, Nu-Lev, Bentyl, and Pro-Banthine, can help relieve the pain of stomach cramping. Side effects of antispasmodics include decreased ability to relieve body heat through sweating, constipation, and dryness of the mouth, nose, throat, or skin.

Lotronex

Experts have found the prescription drug Lotronex (alosetron) to be effective for women experiencing IBS with diarrhea, including stomach pain, distress, and urgency. Lotronex works to block the effect of serotonin on the digestive system.

The role serotonin plays in the development of IBS is uncertain, but researchers do know that Lotronex somehow calms down the colon and slows down the frequency of bowel movements. However, in 2001 the Food and Drug Administration (FDA) took Lotronex off the market, due to its high risk of side effects. As of March 2002 the FDA recorded at least 84 cases of ischemic colitis and 113 cases of serious complications of constipation (needing hospitalization) in connection with Lotronex. The severe side effects of this drug resulted in four deaths. Yet Lotronex had gained strong support among doctors and patients who saw its value in treating the diarrhea associated with IBS. Because of this, in June 2002, the FDA reintroduced the drug, but with several restrictions. Doctors now need to be enrolled in a special program in order to prescribe Lotronex. The drug is approved only for women with severe diarrhea-predominant IBS who have not responded to other treatments.

Imodium and Lomotil

These two drugs are the most common antidiarrhea medications for IBS. They enhance intestinal water absorption, strengthen anal sphincter tone, and decrease intestinal transit, thereby increasing stool consistency and reducing frequency of elimination. Both are intended to be used for the prevention of diarrhea by taking them prior to events (meals or stress) that typically trigger symptoms. They should be taken with plenty of fresh water. Imodium can be used as a daily maintenance drug, but Lomotil is chemically related to narcotics and, as such, is not an innocuous drug, so dosage recommendations should be strictly adhered to (especially in children). Lomotil can be habit-forming, and an overdose could be fatal.

Narcotic Analgesics

Narcotic analgesics for IBS are opioid drugs, and they can be highly effective painkillers. One of their chief side effects, constipation, is actually of benefit to some people with IBS. Narcotics also induce a feeling of tranquility and promote drowsiness, both of which can be helpful for relieving stress-related attacks. The chief problem with narcotic drugs is that it is next to impossible to get a doctor to prescribe them. Although there is mounting evidence that these painkillers are not nearly as habit-forming as previously thought, from your doctor's point of view the risks of addiction are still likely to take precedence over your pain.

Zelnorm

This is a newly released drug specifically formulated for IBS constipation in women, but it hasn't been on the market long enough to determine how effective (or safe) it is. Zelnorm is currently only supposed to be prescribed for short-term use. If you're considering taking this drug for IBS constipation, you'll probably find it helpful to get feedback from other Zelnorm users on the IBS Message Boards on the Internet.

Calmactin (Cilansetron)

This drug for diarrhea-predominant IBS is currently undergoing clinical trials.

Visiting Your Doctor

When you visit your doctor you will want to be able to describe your specific symptoms, express your condition precisely to your doctor, determine what the doctor can do to treat your conditions, and understand what you can do to better manage your situation. Your doctor will begin by taking a history and asking for a description of your symptoms, as well as ascertain the possible factors that bring them on or make them better. This discussion will be probably be followed by a physical examination, including diagnostic tests, a diagnosis, and a discussion of treatment options.

Don't be afraid to ask questions; make a list of them before your appointment. As a person who has IBS, you should never feel devalued, ignored, or uncomfortable with your doctor. If you do, or if your concerns are not being met, it might be time to change to another doctor. Your goals are to obtain a diagnosis, understand IBS and your symptoms, and develop a management or treatment plan designed to meet your individual needs.

The course of IBS is highly individualized, and the condition can be challenging to even the most knowledgeable and caring doctor, so you need to be organized when you go to your appointment. Here are some things you can do to help make your visit to the doctor most effective:

♦ List your symptoms and detail how frequently they occur. Try to be as specific as you can. For example, describe where pain is located, how often it occurs, and what conditions or situtations make it worse or better. Keeping a daily diary for a couple of weeks that lists symptoms and associated activities can help to sort out these aspects. Provide your doctor with a list of all the other chronic illnesses currently affecting your health and detail any prior infectious GI illness. List all of the prescription and nonprescription (over-the-counter) medications you are currently taking, as well as any herbal supplements; include dosages and frequency.

♦ To avoid feeling flustered because of time constraints, jot down a few questions on a notepad before your appointment. Bring the notebook with you and use it to take notes during your appointment. It's imperative that you walk away from your appointment with a clear understanding of what the doctor has told you. Try not to be intimidated by your doctor, and if you have any concerns, such as a fear of cancer, talk about these concerns immediately. In other words, do not hesitate to ask questions. Make sure you understand what your doctor says, and if prescription drugs are suggested as an option, ask if there are alternative options. Don't ever feel pressured into taking drugs.

How Best to Proceed

Your best bet is to find a doctor who understands IBS and who will work with you on monitoring and adapting your individual treatment plan—whether it involves prescription medication or not.

If you do decide to use prescribed prescription drugs, bear in mind that no single drug is approved for all IBS symptoms, and their effectiveness can vary greatly from one person to the next. You and your doctor will have to work together to determine through trial and error which particular drug is best for you. This might take a trial period of a few months and several follow-up visits or phone calls. If you do end up taking a drug and it doesn't work for you, don't feel like you are alone, because many people who have been diagnosed with IBS end up feeling more irritated than relieved after using medications.

Many people with IBS cite great frustration with the lack of safe, reliable, and effective IBS medications on the market, and they would like to see new options be made available to them. Fortunately, there are currently numerous studies and trials underway, so keep your fingers crossed and your eyes open for new treatments on the horizon.

Chapter 9

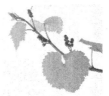

A-to-Z of Specific Symptoms and Natural Ways to Beat Them

Not everyone with IBS is the same. Eating healthily and using the combination of diet and lifestyle changes recommended in *The IBS Healing Plan* that suits you best will help to boost your health, but if you have specific symptoms they can be a special cause of concern. In this chapter you'll learn how to make adjustments and add supplements and power foods, either on their own or with natural therapies, to help you beat your particular symptoms naturally.

Safety First

It's always best to use herbs under the care of a health-care practitioner who is familiar with herbal medicine. Always inform your doctor about all the supplements or herbal medicines you are taking. If you have a history of cardiovascular disease, diabetes, or glaucoma, are pregnant (or hoping to be), or are taking medication, use herbs and supplements only after consulting with your doctor.

The common symptoms of IBS discussed in this chapter include the following:

– Abdominal pain	– Anxiety
– Bloating	– Constipation
– Depression/low mood	– Diarrhea
– Fatigue	– Headaches
– Heartburn	– Nausea

– Cyclical symptoms of IBS
– Gas and gurgling stomach noises

(Note: If fecal incontinence is one of your symptoms, see Chapter 10, "Living with IBS.")

Abdominal Pain

Pain is a defining feature of IBS. Most people can tolerate the diarrhea and constipation, but when they also have to deal with gripping pain and spasms, they can't cope so easily. Pain from spasms can trigger continual bouts of diarrhea and/or constipation. A build-up of gas can also cause pain, as sensitive areas are stretched and twisted. Be guided by your doctor, but there are some things you can do to help ease the pain when it strikes, including the following:

♦ Place a hot water bottle or microwave-heated bag of wheat hulls on your abdomen.

♦ Soak in a warm bath, taking care not to scald yourself.

♦ Drink plenty of clear fluids, such as water, and reduce your intake of coffee, tea, and alcohol because they can make the pain worse.

♦ Try over-the-counter antacids to help reduce some types of pain.

♦ Take mild painkillers, such as acetaminophen (Tylenol). Please check the packet for the right dose. Avoid aspirin or anti-inflammatory drugs unless you have been advised by a doctor to take them. These drugs can worsen some types of abdominal pain.

♦ ♦ ♦

Regular exercise is one of the best ways to decrease your risk of abdominal pain, because exercise releases chemicals called endorphins, which block pain signals in your brain. It's pretty difficult to get morphine, but you have a ready-made supply of endorphins waiting to be released. It's far better to exercise than to find a drug dealer!

Certain types of chronic abdominal discomfort can, in some cases, be eased with pain-management methods, such as biofeedback, cognitive-behavioral therapy, stress management, hypnosis, acupuncture, or acupressure.

Healing herbs for the relief of abdominal pain include ginger, anise, fennel, oregano, peppermint oil, chamomile, and skullcap.

Essential oils derived from geranium, chamomile, neroli, thyme, tea tree, lavender, melissa, petitgrain, peppermint, ginger, and cinnamon leaf are used traditionally as pain relievers for abdominal pain. Put ten to twelve drops of any one of these essential oils in one ounce of a carrier oil, such as olive or coconut. Shake well and then rub into the abdominal area.

(See also the sections on bloating, heartburn, and gas presented later in this chapter, and see the section on stress management in Chapter 6.)

Anxiety

Anxiety is a complex condition that has been described as a feeling of uneasiness in varying degrees. This condition has many facets, and it can be mild to extreme in intensity. Fear of an IBS attack can trigger anxiety, but just living life can produce anxiety for some people. In fact, anxiety can be a forerunner to depressive illnesses and should be treated as soon as possible. In the early stages, the necessity to take the normal drugs prescribed by doctors for anxiety might be avoided by trying some of the following diet and lifestyle changes, as well as herbal alternatives:

♦ Take time out for yourself when you feel anxious. Create your own special place where you can be alone and be free from responsibilities. Write down your feelings in a journal.

♦ Swings in blood sugar can trigger panic and anxiety, so make sure you follow *The IBS Healing Plan* diet guidelines outlined in Chapter 4 and eat little and often to stabilize both your blood sugar levels and your mood.

♦ It is advisable to avoid tranquilizers, antidepressants, alcohol, cocaine, and opium, because these drugs can lead to dependence.

♦ Motherwort contains alkaloids, tannins, and saponins, which act as antispasmodics to calm the heart and nerves without causing sedation.

♦ Passionflower is known to have sedative and analgesic properties, and it has a calming and restful effect on the central nervous system.

♦ Valerian root also affects the central nervous system; it has been used extensively in Europe as a sedative and calmative.

♦ Chamomile is commonly and successfully used for the treatment of anxiety and insomnia, in addition to easing indigestion and GI inflammations. Caraway is also helpful.

♦ Catnip and peppermint also have a sedative effect on the nerves. Lemon balm (*Melissa officinalis*) and common lavender (*Lavandula angustifolia*) are two other herbs that have been shown to be effective in reducing anxiety. Any good naturopath will be able to assist you in obtaining these herbs and the recommended dosages.

♦ The slow movements and controlled postures of yoga improve muscle strength, flexibility, range of motion, balance, breathing, and blood circulation. They also promote mental focus, clarity, and calmness. Stretching also reduces mental and physical stress, tension, and anxiety; promotes good sleep; lowers blood pressure; and slows down your heart rate.

◆ The essential oils that are useful in the treatment of anxiety are bergamot, chamomile, neroli, ylang ylang, melissa, frankincense, cedarwood, lavender, valerian, rose, and vetiver.

◆ Listening to your favorite music is a great way to reduce stress and relieve anxiety. Your individual preferences will determine which type of soothing sounds will best reduce your tension and promote feelings of tranquility. Pay attention to how you feel when you hear a particular song or genre of music, and keep listening to the types that produce a relaxing effect.

◆ Optimism can counteract the negative impact that stress, tension, and anxiety have on your immune system and well-being. Often it is how you perceive things that determines whether you become overwhelmed, both mentally and physically. Having a positive attitude, finding the good in what life throws your way, and looking at the bright side of things enhances your ability to effectively manage stress.

◆ Relaxing in a hot bath relieves sore muscles and joints, reduces stress and tension, and promotes a good night's sleep. Add some soothing music, soft lighting, and naturally scented bath salts or bubble bath/bath foam to create an inexpensive and convenient spa experience in the privacy of your own home.

◆ Relaxation techniques, such as meditation and massage, can promote tranquility and ease anxiety; they might be worth trying out on a regular basis.

ANTIANXIETY FOODS

- *B vitamins.* Women who are depressed or anxious tend to have lower levels of Vitamin B-6, which is needed for the production of serotonin, the brain chemical that lifts mood. Low levels of vitamin B-12 and folic acid can also cause anxiety. To boost your B vitamins, eat plenty of oily fish, eggs, nuts, seeds, soybeans, bananas, and leafy green vegetables.
- *Selenium-rich foods.* People who are deficient in the antioxidant mineral selenium often experience feelings of depression and anxiety. Selenium is found in lean meat, fish, shellfish, Brazil nuts, grains (see advice on eating whole grains in Chapter 4), and avocados.
- *Zinc-rich foods.* Zinc is essential for the body to convert tryptophan into serotonin, the feel-good chemical that can induce feelings of calmness. Zinc is found in eggs, nuts, seeds, peanuts, and sunflower seeds.
- *Oily fish.* Not only does eating oily fish reduce your risk of getting Alzheimer's disease, but according to studies reported in 2003 by the U.S. National Institutes of Health, it reduces anxiety and depression as well.
- *Nuts and seeds.* A handful of nuts and seeds eaten thirty minutes before a potentially stressful situation can help lower anxiety levels by boosting the production of serotonin—that same feel-good chemical we have mentioned a number of times.

Bloating

Over-the-counter remedies to relieve bloating are not advised because they can leach valuable nutrients from your body, but if you have fluid retention as an IBS symptom, there are a number of things you can do to help yourself:

- Cut down on your salt intake. Use less salt in your cooking, watch out for hidden salts in your food, and look for other ways to enhance flavor; for example, by using herbs and spices instead.

♦ Increase your fluid intake. You need to drink more, not less, to help your body dilute the salt in your tissues and allow you to excrete more salt and fluid. Aim to drink at least two quarts of water a day.

♦ Reduce the amount of caffeine in your diet. Caffeine is a diuretic, but it won't ease bloating because it hinders the removal of excess salt and toxins from your body.

♦ Make sure your diet includes sufficient B vitamins, especially vitamin B-6, which is found in bananas, lean meat, fish, and nuts and seeds. This is a tried and tested remedy for water retention.

♦ Eat foods that naturally decrease fluid retention, such as asparagus, cider vinegar, alfalfa sprouts, and dandelion flowers. Eat more potassium-rich food to bring down your body's sodium level (the two minerals counteract one another). so reach for those bananas, apricots, black beans, lentils, tomatoes, green leafy vegetables, and fresh fruits. Keep your blood sugar levels in balance. When blood sugar levels drop, adrenaline is released to move sugar quickly from your cells into your blood. When the sugar leaves the cells, it is replaced by water, and this contributes to that bloated feeling.

♦ Get moving. Moderate exercise will make you sweat and hasten the transport of water through your body.

♦ Studies have shown the surprising effectiveness of Colladeen, a mix of grapeseed extract, bilberry, and cranberry extract, for the relief of bloating.

♦ Dandelion and parsley are natural herbal diuretics packed with hormone-balancing nutrients that allow fluid to be released without losing nutrients.

♦ Bloating is often caused by intestinal gas, which can result from swallowing air or eating gas-producing foods. Swallowing air while eating is often done unconsciously and might

FOOD PRODUCTS THAT ALLEVIATE BLOATING

- *Olive oil.* This useful oil promotes the overall absorption of nutrients and helps the digestive system function more efficiently. It can help reduce bloating because it is very well tolerated by the stomach due to its high oleic acid content. The sphincter that separates the stomach from the esophagus is less affected by olive oil than any other fat—which means less indigestion, less acidity, and less bloating. Taking two tablespoonfuls of olive oil in the morning on an empty stomach also appears to have a positive effect on chronic constipation, another cause of bloating.

- *Soy yogurt. Lactobacillus acidophilus* is one of the friendly bacteria that live in the intestines. When eaten, it travels to the intestines and crowds out the harmful bacteria that might be causing painful gas and bloating. One source of these bacteria is yogurt that contains live, active culture. It's important to look for yogurts that specifically say they contain live culture, because many types of yogurts are heat-treated to kill the bacteria before being sold. For people who either can't tolerate dairy products or who choose not to eat dairy products, a number of very tasty soy-based yogurts are currently available at many health-food stores.

- *Fiber.* Throughout the day, snack on other high-fiber foods like strawberries, blueberries, dried apricots, and dried plums. But be careful that you don't add too much fiber too quickly, or you'll feel even more bloated than before. Your body needs time to get used to processing the increased bulk.

- *Bananas.* Bloating can also be relieved by increasing your intake of vitamin B-6, which is a natural diuretic. Healthy foods that are rich in vitamin B-6 include bananas, alfalfa, lentils, oily fish, soy products, raw nuts and seeds (especially walnuts), rye, turkey, oats, brown rice, and green leafy vegetables.

- *Fennel tea.* You also might want to try fennel tea. Brew a tablespoonful or so of fennel in a tea strainer and drink several cups a day. Fennel tastes like licorice and has antigas and antispasmodic properties, making it especially helpful in relieving bloating. It's also a very safe herbal remedy that you can use daily without any risks.

result in frequent belching during or after meals. To avoid swallowing air, slow down when eating, don't "slurp" drinks, and don't talk while chewing. Also try to avoid chewing gum, hard sweets, carbonated drinks (such as soda pop), and drinking through straws.

♦ Aromatherapy oils can be helpful in relieving bloating. Add fennel or chamomile to a warm bath and soak for twenty minutes for the best effect. You might also want to use juniper as a massage oil.

(Note: If the abdomen is tender to the touch or hard, contact your doctor to make sure that there is not a more serious underlying cause for the bloating. Although uncommon, bloating can also be caused by ovarian cancer and ascites, which is the presence of excess fluid often associated with liver disease and also sometimes with cancer.)

Constipation

Sometimes nothing's moving, even though you know you have to move your bowels. You might even feel as if you are ready to empty your bowels. Everything in your body is sending you this signal. You feel bloated and have uncomfortable pressure, but when you try to go, nothing happens, or if you do finally go, it hurts.

It's not a good idea to use laxatives as the first line of attack when you're constipated. They can become habit-forming to the point that they damage your colon. Some laxatives can inhibit the effectiveness of medications you might be taking, and there are laxatives that cause inflammation to the lining of the intestines. If you must take a laxative, find one that is psyllium- or fiber-based. Psyllium is a natural fiber that's much gentler on the system than the ingredients in many of the other products available today.

Bump up your fiber intake by switching from refined foods to natural foods whenever possible. Switch from a highly processed cereal to a whole-grain cereal, move from heavily cooked vegetables to lightly cooked or raw vegetables, and choose whole-grain products over products made with white flour. Sometimes, a little extra dietary fiber is all you need to ensure regularity. Fiber is found naturally in fruits, vegetables, grains, and beans (although refining and processing can significantly decrease the fiber content of these products). To avoid getting gas, increase the fiber in your diet gradually, and be sure you drink plenty of water so the fiber can move smoothly through your digestive system. (See also the advice on soluble and insoluble fiber in Chapter 4, "Healing IBS with Diet.") Try taking a teaspoonful of linseed in the morning and another in the evening; chew the linseed thoroughly or grind it just before eating.

Here are some further dietary tips you might find helpful:

+ *Blackstrap molasses.* When necessary, take two tablespoonfuls before going to bed to relieve constipation. Molasses is too high in calories to use as a daily preventative, but on an occasional basis it can help get your bowels to move. It has a pretty strong taste, so you might want to add it to milk, fruit juice, or, for an extra-powerful laxative punch, prune juice.

+ *Walnuts.* Eaten fresh from the shell, these might be just the laxative you need.

+ *Beans.* Dried beans and legumes, whether they're pinto beans, red beans, lima beans, black beans, navy beans, or garbanzo beans, are excellent sources of fiber. Many people don't like them because they can give you gas. Cooking beans properly, however, can ease this problem considerably. Soak them first, discard the soaking water, and then add ginger, cumin, or fennel seeds to the beans in a new pot of cooking water. Make sure they are quite soft before you eat them. Plus, if you add beans to your diet gradually, you'll minimize the effects of any gas they might produce.

+ *Oregon grape.* The root of this plant has been used safely since ancient times to overcome occasional constipation. Mix half a teaspoonful of Oregon grape tincture in water and sip slowly before eating for best results.

+ *Fruit and vegetables.* Eat at least five servings of fruit and vegetables daily. Eat an apple one hour after a meal to prevent constipation. Apple juice and apple cider are also natural laxatives for some people. Bananas can ease constipation, too. Try eating two ripe bananas between meals, but avoid green bananas because they can actually cause constipation. Ttry a handful of raisins an hour after a meal. Rhubarb is also a natural laxative.

♦ *Sesame seeds.* These seeds provide roughage and bulk, and they soften the contents of the intestines, which makes elimination easier. Eat no more than one-half ounce daily, and drink lots of water while consuming them.

♦ *Garlic.* Eaten raw, garlic has a laxative effect for many people. Eat it mixed with onion, raw or cooked, or with milk or yogurt for best results.

♦ *Hot water with lemon.* Drink a cup first thing in the morning before you eat breakfast to help get things moving.

♦ *Honey.* This is a very mild laxative. Try taking one tablespoonful three times a day, either by itself or mixed into warm water.

♦ *Safflower, soybean, or other vegetable oils.* These can be just the cure you need because they provide a lubricating effect in the intestines. Take two to three tablespoonfuls a day, but use only until the problem is gone (i.e., not on an ongoing, everyday basis). If you don't like taking oil straight from the spoon, mix the oil with herbs and lemon juice or vinegar to use as a salad dressing. The combination of the oil and the fiber from the salad will likely relieve your constipation.

♦ *Vinegar.* Mix one teaspoonful of cider vinegar and one teaspoonful of honey in a glass of water and drink.

Although your diet is likely to be the primary thing you need to change in order to relieve constipation, there are other lifestyle changes that can also help. Stress, certain medications, and lack of exercise may be the culprit. Exercise, in particular, boosts regularity. When you are active, so are your bowels—so the more sedentary you are, the more slowly your bowels will move. Here are some other tips:

+ *Heed the call.* People sometimes suppress the urge to have a bowel movement because they are busy or have an erratic schedule, or because they don't want to use public bathrooms. If at all possible, heed the call when you feel it.

+ *Don't rush.* It takes time for your bowels to move, so allow sufficient time and be patient. It *will* happen. If you feel the urge but can't manage a bowel movement, avoid pushing and straining, and perform the colonic massage technique listed below several times a day instead.

COLONIC MASSAGE

Perform this massage either while sitting on the toilet or lying down with your knees bent. Make a fist with your right hand and massage your colon using a digging, circular motion with your knuckles. Start at the lower right quadrant of your abdomen (just inside your hip bone) and work up to under the right side of your rib cage, then straight across, then down the left quadrant of your abdomen. When you get to just inside your left hipbone, massage inward toward your groin/pubic bone. The idea is to massage the length of your colon. This starts at the lower-right quadrant of your abdomen, and then proceeds up in a horseshoe shape under the ribs and down to the lower-left quadrant of your abdomen. The rectal canal then extends from the lower-left quadrant diagonally across to the groin (or pubic bone). Repeat the massage several times, experimenting with varying pressure. This is a fantastic technique that can be used by anyone either during a bowel movement, or to encourage the bowels to move. This massage technique also relieves colic in newborn babies by helping them to expel gas and stools.

Cyclical Symptoms of IBS

Many women notice that their IBS symptoms worsen around the time of their period. This occurs because when a woman's period

starts, levels of the hormones estrogen and progesterone drop naturally, and this shift can trigger diarrhea, gas, bloating, and pain.

Women with IBS have symptoms all month, but their symptoms
can get worse the week before their period. This means their IBS
symptoms can become jumbled up with the PMS symptoms of bloating, anxiety, food cravings, breast tenderness, and mood swings, and
their diarrhea symptoms often become more pronounced during
their period. Thus, it is easy to confuse period pains and cramps with
the symptoms of IBS. If you find that your IBS symptoms become
more pronounced before or around your period, you can use this
information to your advantage. For example, you can make plans to
deal with both your IBS symptoms and your period problems, based
on your knowledge of your menstrual cycle (e.g., it might be a good
idea to avoid air travel or important meetings in the middle of your
period.).

There are a number of natural ways to ease PMS, and the most
common ones are listed below. In general you will find that the steps
recommended in *The IBS Healing Plan* to ease your IBS symptoms
will also help ease any symptoms of PMS.

- *Change your diet.* Eat little and often, and choose foods that
  are rich in fiber. This will help to stabilize your blood sugar
  and ease mood swings, anxiety, depression, and fatigue.
  Reducing your intake of salt and caffeine can help decrease
  water retention and ease breast tenderness. Taking steps to
  avoid constipation can also help some women (see the advice
  in the previous section). Make sure sure you drink enough
  water (paradoxically, this also helps to ease fluid retention).

- *Take a dietary supplement.* Calcium and magnesium can help
  balance your hormones and keep you calm. Vitamin B-6
  aids serotonin production. Several commercial PMS formu-
  las contain these and other beneficial ingredients. Evening
  primrose oil is especially helpful for breast tenderness.

- *Try Vitex agnus-castus.* A number of studies have shown
  that this ancient herbal remedy can help reduce mental

and physical symptoms in up to 90 percent of women. Vitex agnus-castus works on the pituitary gland to regulate the production of hormones. Give it time, though, because it can take up to three months to work.

♦ *Do some gentle exercise.* Gentle exercise, like swimming or yoga, releases the brain chemicals (endorphins) that make us feel happy, more alert, and less anxious. Try to exercise throughout the month, but if you exercise when PMS is at its worst, you should receive some immediate relief.

Depression/Low Mood

Everyone gets sad from time to time, and having a chronic condition like IBS can wear down optimism and enthusiasm. If your mood is persistently low, however, it's important to seek advice from your doctor to discover the underlying cause. If IBS is dragging you down, the following natural mood-boosters might help.

A "Positive Voice"

In 2002 researchers in England found that a person's perception of their bowel disorder affects how they cope with the condition. If they think optimistically about their condition and their life they cope well, but if they think negatively, the symptoms are often worse. If you analyze your thoughts you might be surprised at how negative they are. For example, if you drop something you might think, "Gosh, I'm stupid." If you bump into someone you might think, "Why am I so clumsy?" If you're struggling with your weight you might think, "I'm fat and ugly." Try to catch yourself every time you have a negative thought about yourself or the things you do— and counter that thought with one that is more positive or realistic. If you drop something or make a mistake, try: "Okay, I messed up, but what about all the times when I've gotten things right," or "I was looking where I was going; the other person wasn't." If you feel very brave, go for, "That wasn't my fault."

List the Positive

List all the good things in your life. These things might be a job you enjoy, a loyal friend, a fascinating hobby, your dog, the flowers in your garden, and so on. Now make a list of all the good things about yourself. Think this over carefully, because there is bound to be a lot more than you realized. You might be a good listener or a great poet or have a great sense of humor.

Find New Challenges

Taking on a new challenge can be incredibly rewarding and can make you feel more positive about yourself. If you've always wanted to learn how to play the piano or keyboard, arrange for some lessons. Or take up painting, singing, jewelry-making, or writing—the list is endless. Or perhaps you might like to get some new qualifications or take a course, or even study a subject that is helpful in dealing with IBS, such as homeopathy, reflexology, massage, and so on.

Physical Activity

Physical activity can contribute greatly to a sense of well-being. In fact, regular exercise is considered by some experts to be one of the most effective treatments for depression. Plan to do at least thirty minutes of gentle exercise a day.

Everyday Boosters

Sing along to your favorite music, have a good cry to release excess stress, and enjoy a boisterous laugh. Laughter sends endorphins, which we've mentioned before, whizzing around your body to make you feel naturally high. So do something to get you chuckling—anything from watching a funny film to phoning an old friend.

St. John's Wort

This herb has been shown in numerous studies to demonstrate a significant improvement in depression, anxiety, and insomnia. It's taken in daily doses of 2–4 grams, calculated to contain 0.2–1.0 milligrams of hypericin, the active ingredient. Capsules containing 300 milligrams of the extract (and 0.3 percent hypericin) are typically taken three times a day. However, you should consult your doctor if you are considering taking St. John's wort to be sure it is safe for *you* to take.

Ginger

Ginger has been a powerhouse in Traditional Chinese Medicine for thousands of years. It is an herb that decreases fatigue and weakness, and it is potentially valuable for combating depression. It is also helpful for digestion and acts as an anti-inflammatory.

Bach Flower Remedies

Wild rose, larch, mustard, gorse, and gentian help to alleviate feelings of apathy, resignation, despondency, inferiority, despair, hopelessness, discouragement, self-doubt, and intense descending gloom.

Sunlight

Sunlight is vital for both physical and emotional health. Try to get fifteen minutes of sunlight on your uncovered eyelids daily (remove your glasses and take out your contact lenses) in the early morning or late afternoon. In the absence of sun, try sitting next to six to eight regular fluorescent tubes (2,500 lux) for thirty minutes each day upon waking.

Massage

Massage is often more effective than talk therapy for uncovering and healing hidden traumas and relieving depression. Even a single session can have a dramatic effect.

Posture

Stand tall, smile with your whole face, and breathe deeply. You will either start to feel happier or make your rage/grief more visible and more easily accessed.

Sigh!

To energize yourself when depressed, you can sigh deeply many times, hold your arms out in front of you for several minutes, or bounce up and down on the balls of your feet. Try it!

A healthy diet rich in whole grains, fruits, vegetables, legumes, nuts, seeds, and oily fish is the foundation of a diet to beat depression. The following foods are so rich in nutrients that can boost mood that they deserve special mention.

FOODS THAT FIGHT DEPRESSION

- *Grapefruit.* This is great for boosting liver function and easing depression. The more toxins your liver is exposed to, the more easily its detoxification systems are overloaded. If the liver is sluggish, excessive amounts of toxins find their way into the bloodstream, which can affect the function of the brain, causing unpleasant and erratic mood changes, a general feeling of depression, "foggy brain," and an impaired ability to concentrate or remember things.

- *Artichoke.* This is liver protective, and it also has a bile-producing and bile-moving effect on the liver. When bile lingers in the liver, it irritates the tissue, creating inflammation and decreasing the ability of the liver to carry out its functions, so you are more likely to feel tired and depressed.

- *Watermelon.* Studies indicate that red-pigmented, lycopene-rich foods such as tomatoes, papaya, and watermelon improve liver health, and a healthy liver is essential for detoxification and physical, emotional, mental health and general well-being.

- *Sunflower seeds.* Minerals are essential for the growth and functioning of the brain. Selenium (high levels are also found in seafood and seaweed), which is found in sunflower seeds, has been shown to improve mood significantly. Other sources of selenium include Brazil nuts, tuna, and whole-grain cereals.

(cont'd.)

- *Oily fish/linseed.* Fatty acids regulate memory and mood. The brain is made up of 60 percent fatty acids. The omega-3 types (DHA and EPA) are essential for the optimal performance of your brain. Omega fatty acids are found in oily fish—for example, mackerel, tuna, herring, salmon, and sardines, as well as other foods, such as avocados, olives, raw nuts and seeds, and their cold-pressed oils. All of the aforementioned foods contain good mood stimulants, and it has been discovered that levels of depression can be improved by introducing the healthy fats these foods provide into your diet. Omega-3 oils are also excellent for boosting intelligence and memory. If you don't eat fish, try consuming hemp or linseed oils instead.

- *Lentils.* These are an excellent source of B vitamins and folate. Folate deficiency has been linked to an increased risk of depression, and a deficiency in B vitamins increases the risk of anxiety, insomnia, and mood swings.

- *Water.* The body deteriorates rapidly without water, and dehydration is a common cause of tiredness, poor concentration, and reduced alertness. So make sure you get your recommended eight glasses a day!

Diarrhea

If you frequently suffer from diarrhea, try to avoid taking any anti-diarrhea medications until you have given *The IBS Healing Plan* recommendations and the suggestions described below a chance to work. Acute diarrhea is a common short-term problem that usually resolves on its own, and chronic long-term diarrhea, as a symptom of IBS, responds well to dietary modifications.

In order to help restore balance in your body, try consuming potassium-rich bananas, apple sauce, and dry toast until you feel better. You can also use live yogurt to replace any beneficial bacteria in your intestines that may have been lost through diarrhea. Here are some other suggestions:

- ♦ *Blueberries.* Blueberry root is a long-time folk remedy for diarrhea. In Sweden, doctors prescribe a soup made with dried blueberries for tummy problems. Blueberries are rich

in anthocyanosides, which have antioxidant and antibacterial properties, as well as tannins, which combat diarrhea.

♦ *Chamomile tea.* Chamomile is good for treating intestinal inflammation, and it has antispasmodic properties as well. You
can brew yourself a cup of chamomile tea from packaged
teabags, or you can buy chamomile flowers and steep one
teaspoonful of them and one teaspoonful of peppermint
leaves in a cup of boiling water for fifteen minutes. Drink
three cups a day.

♦ *Potatoes.* This is another starchy food that can help to restore both nutrients and comfort to your stomach. However,
eating French fries won't help because fried foods tend to
aggravate an aching tummy. Other root vegetables, such as
carrots (cooked, of course), are also easy on an upset stomach, and they are loaded with nutrients.

♦ *Bananas.* Long known as a soother for tummy troubles,
this potassium-rich fruit can restore nutrients and is easy
to digest.

♦ *Orange peel.* Orange peel tea is a folk remedy that is believed
to aid in digestion. Place a chopped orange peel (preferably
from an organic orange to avoid possible pesticides and
dyes) into a pot and cover with one pint of boiling water.
Let it stand until the water is cooled. You can sweeten the
tea with sugar or honey.

♦ *L-glutamine.* This amino acid is another remedy for diarrhea.
For some people it works very quickly (within two to three
days, usually). It's virtually tasteless and dissolves easily in
water. Start with one-fourth of a teaspoonful per day mixed
into cold or room-temperature water and drink it on an
empty stomach. If that's not enough, increase to one-fourth
of a teaspoonful two or three times a day. Then increase the
dosage gradually (if you need it) to one-half teaspoonful,
then three-fourths of a teaspoonful, and finally up to one

teaspoonful two or three times a day. L-glutamine directly nourishes and heals the mucosal lining of the intestines and causes the bowel to reabsorb the water in your stools, thus reducing the number and frequency of bowel movements. *Note: Do not use L-glutamine if you have a liver or kidney disease.*

◆ *Avoid diarrhea-causing foods.* These include refined sugar, re-fined flour (white, bleached), hydrogenated fats, caffeine, and acidic, tomato-based foods, such as spaghetti sauce and pizza. Most people find coffee (regular or decaffeinated) highly ir-ritating as well. Anyone with IBS should automatically avoid processed foods, luncheon meats and hot dogs, and foods containing artificial flavors/color, preservatives, or MSG.

◆ *Colonic massage.* This is also an excellent way to reduce the frequency of bowel movements because massage helps to move all the separate little stool deposits around the colon and out at once, rather than in numerous separate bowel movements (see "Colonic Massage" on page 111).

◆ *Keep hydrated.* You can lose large amounts of liquid during bouts of diarrhea, and you also lose electrolytes, minerals such as sodium and potassium that are critical in the proper functioning of your body. So make sure you drink plenty of fluids. Whatever you choose to drink, keep it cool; it will be less irritating that way. Sip, don't guzzle; it will be easier on your insides if you take frequent sips of liquid instead of guz-zling down a glass at a time.

◆ *Cut out caffeine.* Just as it stimulates your nervous system, caffeine jump-starts your intestines. And that's the last thing you need when you have diarrhea.

◆ *Say "NO" to sweet treats.* High concentrations of sugar can exacerbate diarrhea. The sugar in fruit can do the same. Steer clear of greasy or high-fiber foods. These are harder for your gut to handle. You need foods that are kind and gentle.

In short, stick as much as possible to the recommendations for diet in Chapter 4, "Healing IBS with Diet."

Although usually not harmful, diarrhea can become dangerous or signal a more serious problem. You should see the doctor if—

♦ you have diarrhea for more than three days

♦ you have severe pain in the abdomen or rectum

♦ you have a fever of 102 degrees Fahrenheit or higher

♦ you see blood in your stools or have black, tarry stools

♦ you have signs of dehydration—headaches, thirst, fatigue, or dark yellow urine

(Note: If your child has diarrhea, do not hesitate to call the doctor for advice. Diarrhea can be dangerous in children if too much fluid is lost and not replaced quickly.)

Fatigue

Tiredness and fatigue are often reported by people with IBS. All the natural therapies suggested in this book should help boost your energy levels, but the following suggestions might be particularly helpful:

♦ Make sure you balance out your carbohydrate load with some low-fat protein to avoid the sugar highs and lows that cause fatigue. In fact, balancing your blood sugar levels is the best way to fight fatigue and boost your energy levels.

♦ Step up your exercise routine; people who exercise regularly tend to feel more energized than people who do not.

♦ Eat foods that are high in fatigue-fighting potassium and magnesium. Prime sources include fruit, green leafy vegetables, nuts, seeds, and beans. You also need to make sure you are getting enough iron-rich foods, including wheat germ, dried fruit, shellfish, sardines, and red and dark-green fruits and vegetables. If you are a vegetarian, you might want to take kelp supplements.

♦ The B vitamins are crucial if you feel tired, because one of the symptoms of a deficiency of the major B vitamins is lack of energy.

♦ Co-enzyme Q10 (CoQ10), a substance present in all human tissue, is a vital catalyst for energy production, and if you are deficient in this enzyme you might feel tired. Food sources of CoQ10 include fish, organ meats (like liver, heart, or kidney), and the germ portion of whole grains. You might also want to take 30 milligrams a day of CoQ10 supplement over a period of three months.

♦ Ginger can boost energy levels. Use it fresh in your food for a quick pick-me-up. Cinnamon is another energy-boosting spice.

♦ Aromatherapy oils, such as basil and rosemary, can be helpful in treating mental and physical fatigue. Both are stimulating and renewing, and you might want to add a few drops to your bath or use them in a vaporizer in your room.

Refer to the recommendations for stress-busting and getting a good night's sleep that are in Chapter 7, "Healing IBS with Stress Management," because both stress and lack of sleep can cause fatigue.

If your fatigue persists, you might want to rule out conditions of hypertension, diabetes, candida, thyroid problems, anemia, and/or a food allergy. Consult your doctor.

Gas and Gurgling Stomach Noises

Burping and breaking wind are the ways in which the body rids itself of swallowed air, so you can cut down on unwanted and potentially embarrassing burps by reducing how much air you swallow. Here are some suggestions to promote this relief:

♦ *Stifle it.* Sometimes burping and breaking wind produce such an inordinate sense of relief that chronic burping will encourage a person to burp even more. It's better not to do this, because repeated burping can trigger more burping.

♦ *Don't smoke.* Here is yet another reason to stop smoking. When you inhale smoke from cigarettes, cigars, or pipes, you swallow excessive amounts of air.

♦ *Watch what you put in your mouth.* Chewing gum and sucking on hard sweets or lollipops stimulates air swallowing.

♦ *Mind your manners.* Avoid talking with your mouth full, because this makes you swallow air, and the more air you swallow the more likely you are to burp or break wind.

♦ *Eat slowly.* People who gulp down food and drinks swallow excessive amounts of air. This also crowds the stomach with too much to digest, which causes the build-up of gas.

♦ *Limit your drinking of fizzy drinks.* Drinking carbonated beverages, including beer, creates air in the stomach, which has to come out one way or another.

♦ *Relax.* Anxiety and stress can cause you to swallow more often, which increases the amount of air taken in. When you feel stressed, force yourself to breathe slowly and deeply.

♦ *Don't use straws.* Drinking through a straw increases the amount of air that you swallow.

♦ *Stay active.* Don't lie down after you eat. Activity will force the burps and gas out of your system instead of letting them build up.

♦ *Keep a diary.* Keep a diary, noting foods and beverages consumed, as well as specific incidents prior to the start of burping. You might discover that you are more burp- or gas-prone immediately after you eat certain foods, such as dairy products.

♦ *Ginger tea.* This tea can help relieve the need to burp or pass gas. Lemon juice might also help. Papaya is full of an enzyme called *papain,* which might get rid of whatever is causing your gas. Peppermint and other herbs (carminatives) that soothe the digestive tract might also ease belching and decrease bloating after large meals.

If you are worried about the smell created by breaking wind, refer to the section on fecal incontinence in Chapter 10, "Living with IBS."

Gurgling Stomach Noises

Stomach noises can get quite loud, causing social embarrassment. You might be able to laugh it off with friends, but it's another thing altogether when it happens during a critical business meeting. To describe stomach noises, doctors use the word *borborygmi,* which basically means the sounds that come from your digestive system as food, air, and gas move through your body. If your stomach is trying to get your attention and you're tired of the turmoil, try the following tips:

♦ *Sip some warm ginger ale.* Warm ginger ale might be just what the doctor ordered for a gurgling stomach, provided the gurgles are caused by gas or air. Putting soda bubbles in your belly can encourage any gas trapped in your stomach to come up as a belch so that it's over and done with.

♦ *Sneak a snack.* Stomachs gurgle more when they are empty, so if you eat regular meals and snacks the problem can be avoided. If you don't have time for a meal, sneaking a snack should silence your stomach. If you're in a hurry, try eating a cracker or a piece of bread, which might stop the noises from occurring.

♦ *Don't gulp.* Have you ever tried to take a deep breath to stop your stomach from gurgling? You might have made the situation worse. You're just taking in more air, which was part of

the problem in the first place. So if you do take a deep breath
or yawn, try not to swallow the air.

Headaches

Missing meals or nutrients can trigger a headache whether you have
IBS or not, so make sure you don't allow more than a few hours between meals and snacks.

See if you can find a pattern or a trigger to your headaches.
When you get a headache, note what you ate, when you ate, and
how you felt when you ate. Perhaps you are sensitive to certain foods.
Watch out especially for foods such as cheese, red wine, chocolate,
citrus juice or fruits that contain tyramine, phenylethylamine, and
histamine, all of which can trigger headaches. Unfortunately, symptoms often don't hit you immediately after eating these foods, so you
need to keep a diary for several weeks to notice a pattern. Typical
tension headache triggers include stress, fatigue, too much sleep,
lack of exercise, and activities that require repetitive motion, such
as chewing gum or grinding teeth.

Magnesium helps your muscles relax, and a deficiency can trigger headaches. Make sure your diet includes foods such as leafy
green vegetables, nuts and seeds, dark chocolate, and soybeans.

Also make sure that your diet is rich in essential fatty acids—
especially omega-3. One study showed that people with migraine
have a significant reduction in symptoms when they take omega-3
fish oils every day.

It's best to avoid over-the-counter painkillers because many of
them contain caffeine. Also, you can easily become intolerant to
these drugs.

Learn to relax. You might be able to ward off a fair number of
headaches by reducing muscle tension. Sit or lie down in a dark,
quiet room for twenty minutes and place an ice pack on your forehead (note, though, that some tension headaches respond better to
the application of heat). When headaches or migraines play a part
in your life, try to regard them as evidence that you need time to be

alone, rest, and recharge. Lie in total silence, in complete darkness, and sleep, if possible, until the headache is gone. Regular exercise and stretching can prevent many tension headaches.

Treat yourself to a neck, shoulder, and head massage. Whether using traditional massage or acupressure, releasing physical tension and improving circulation can promote feelings of well-being and even prevent headaches. Simply rubbing your temples can relieve pain.

Putting an ice pack on the area where the pain is focused can reduce the blood flow, which in turn eases the pain. In some cases a warm bath can make people who are prone to headaches feel better, especially if an essential herb such as lavender is added. Other helpful oils include rosemary, which can stimulate blood supply to the head, and eucalyptus, which eases pain. Add a few drops to your bath or make up a massage oil to use with neck and shoulder massage.

Use a blend of relaxing aromatherapy oils as a massage oil or add a few drops in your bath. Lavender, chamomile, and rosemary can all ease pain.

If you have a tension headache and can't get to a dark room to relax, put your hands around the back of your head and drop your chin on your chest. Press your chin down and hold it there for a minute. Then use your hands to turn your head to the right and hold for a minute. Then move your head back to center and hold for a minute, then turn it to the left and then back to center again for a minute.

One study showed that 70 percent of the people who get migraines have less frequent attacks when taking the herb feverfew. Milk thistle might also be beneficial because it helps improve liver function. Other useful herbs include cayenne, chamomile, garden sage, elderflower, ground ivy, Jamaican dogwood, lady's slipper, lavender, marjoram, peppermint, rosemary, rue, skullcap, tansy, thyme, valerian, wood betony, and wormwood.

Don't ignore headaches that occur over and over again. They could be a sign of an underlying health problem. If you have tried various "do-it-yourself" measures with no success or your headaches become more intense or persistent, ask your doctor for advice.

Heartburn

Heartburn is often reported in people with IBS. It is caused by burning stomach acid (generated by digestion) washing back up into the throat. Heartburn is best treated by using a natural approach. You do not really need to spend a lot of money on antacid or reflux medications. There are many home remedies that are very effective in relieving the discomforts brought on by heartburn.

One of the most common ways to treat heartburn is to dilute one tablespoonful of baking soda in a glass of water. For many years, baking soda has been recognized as one of the best solutions to heartburn. The good thing about baking soda is that it's cheap. If you use baking soda to treat heartburn you will not need to spend a lot of money, and you will not need to see your doctor to get a prescription since it is readily available in supermarkets.

According to experts, apples are great acid neutralizers. For many years, people have used the natural antacids found in apples to relieve the discomforts brought about by heartburn. The good thing about apples is that you can eat as many as you like without getting any adverse effects. Because apples are very rich in fiber and vitamins that can help your body to remain healthy and strong, the more apples you eat, the better off you will be.

You need to discover your triggers. If you learn what brings on your heartburn, you can avoid the triggers and eliminate the condition. Avoid acidic foods and drink—for example, tomatoes, oranges, grapefruit, alcohol, and lemons. Also avoid chocolate, peppermint, spearmint, high-fat foods, and caffeine—especially in the evening.

Avoid lying down or reclining for two hours after eating.

Gently massage your esophageal valve by rubbing gently just under your solar plexus and stroking downwards toward your belly button.

When you go to sleep, lie on your left side. Your stomach opens up to your left and this encourages the food and acids to stay in your stomach and away from your esophageal valve.

Herbs that can help prevent heartburn include black pepper, cardamom seed, coriander seed, fennel seed, peppermint leaf, and licorice root.

Nausea

If nausea is one of your common symptoms, try using some of the following natural remedies:

* *Lime juice.* For an immediate nausea stopper, mix one cup of water, ten drops of lime juice, and one-half teaspoonful of sugar. Then add one-fourth teaspoonful of baking soda and drink.

* *Onion.* Juice an onion to make one teaspoonful of liquid. Mix this with one teaspoonful of grated ginger and take for nausea (as long as onion is not one of the foods that triggers your IBS).

* *Anise.* This helps to cure nausea and vomiting. Brew anise into a tea by putting one-fourth teaspoonful in one-half cup of boiling water. Steep for five minutes. Strain and drink once a day. Or sprinkle some anise on mild vegetables, such as cooked carrots or pumpkin.

* *Cinnamon.* For nausea, steep one-half teaspoonful of cinnamon powder in one cup of boiling water, strain, and sip. Do not try this remedy if you're pregnant.

* *Cumin.* Steep a tea with one teaspoonful of cumin seeds and a pinch of nutmeg to soothe tummy troubles.

* *Fennel.* Crush one tablespoonful of seeds and steep for ten minutes in one cup of boiling water. Sweeten to taste with honey. Sip as necessary for nausea.

♦ *Ginger.* Without doubt, ginger is the best stomach-woe cure. Taken in any form, it can relieve nausea. Try ginger tea, gingerbread, or gingersnaps.

♦ *Mint.* Mint tea relieves nausea. Steep one tablespoonful of dry leaves in one pint of hot water for thirty minutes, then strain and drink. Don't toss out those mint leaves when you drink the tea. Instead, eat them. Eating boiled mint leaves can also help cure nausea.

♦ *Acupressure* has been found to be effective for reducing nausea. You can purchase pressure bands in many pharmacies that are to be worn around your wrists; gently and constantly applying pressure to acupuncture points and by so doing easing nausea.

♦ *Chamomile.* If you experience nausea along with digestive distress, try drinking chamomile tea three times a day.

♦ *Vitamin B-6.* This can also help to quell nausea. Increase the amount in your diet by eating foods such as spinach, tuna, banana, and salmon, or take a supplement.

If, in addition to nausea, you experience a loss of appetite and difficulty swallowing, or feel pain when you swallow, you should contact your doctor immediately for advice.

Chapter 10

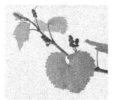

Living with IBS

IBS is a real challenge because it is such an unpredictable medical condition. You might wake up one morning and feel great, and then by lunchtime you are doubled up in agony and have an urgent need to go to the bathroom. It's no surprise, then, that some people with IBS become anxious about even leaving their homes. They might also be afraid to switch jobs, go to a restaurant, travel, or have almost any type of social life because they are worried that their symptoms might flare up when there is no bathroom in sight.

Louis, age 38

It has been about eight or nine years since I was diagnosed with IBS, and it has been nothing but hell for me. Going to work, I have to make sure I know where a toilet is along the route; when going to the store, I go to the bathroom before I leave home, and then I sit in the car because I start to feel light-headed like I'm going to be sick. Being at a party is the worst because of all the people; even at my own parties I feel ill. There have also been embarrassing times where I haven't been able to make it to the toilet in time, and being over thirty, it's not the nicest of feelings when you've soiled yourself. I'm still suffering with IBS, and I would like to one day go into a shopping center with my wife and do some shopping without having all these problems.

Hopefully, the information given in this book about diet, supplements, alternative therapies, stress management, and working
with your doctor will help you feel more confident about your ability
to take charge of your condition, become an active participant in
your own health-care, and live your life to the fullest. However, for
those days when you are scared to leave home in case you can't find
a bathroom, or you dread the mealtimes when you afraid of eating
in case it might trigger an attack, or those moments when you are
worried about ever having a normal bowel movement again and being doomed to a life of misery, the aim of this chapter is to give you
some extra tools and an extra boost of confidence to get you out of
your home and on with your life. (For tips on eating in restaurants,
refer to Chapter 4, "Healing IBS with Diet.")

Fecal Incontinence

If you have fecal incontinence with your IBS—involuntarily breaking wind and losing some of your bowel contents at the same time
—then this is probably one of your most feared events. It really
isn't something you want to talk about with anyone because of the
stigma attached. Following the IBS Healing Plan can certainly help
to ease this symptom, but if it's something you are prone to, then
wearing a small panty liner—the kind women use on light days of
their period—is a great confidence-booster, whether you are a man
or a woman. Panty liners have an adhesive strip that attaches to
your underwear, and they have absorbent material on one side and
plastic on the other to prevent moisture from reaching your underwear. Panty liners are small, thin, and easy to carry with you in a bag
or even your pocket.

If your problem is bigger than the size of a panty liner, never resort to inserting a tampon into your anus or blocking the anus with
a pack of tissues when you go out, because these measures dry up
the secretions your anus needs to stay healthy. Instead, go for adult
diapers or briefs—they come in various shapes and sizes, designed
for light or heavy incontinence. Many adult briefs are disposable,

have absorbent material that neutralizes odors, and provide anti-leak cuffs. If you are embarrassed about buying them at the store, you can always say they are for an elderly relative, or you can order them on the Internet. Okay, they might not look or feel that attractive, but if you want to get back to living your life to the fullest, you need to adapt. The chances are you won't even need them for a long period of time, and wearing them now is just your "security blanket" so you can stop worrying and get on with living.

(Note: In addition to wearing panty liners or a pad, it also makes sense to carry some adult wet wipes and a change of underwear in your bag or purse.)

Covering Up Odors

Are you embarrassed about leaving a bad smell behind, especially at work, in public bathrooms, or in a friend's home? Remember, you aren't alone; everyone experiences this problem at one time or another. If you are concerned about lingering smells, make sure you flush several times and always carry a small can of air freshener in your bag, but don't use fruity-smelling odors because they just make the odor worse. Try to buy a product that kills odors, not masks them. You could also try striking a match in the bathroom. This helps to mask the smell. (Do be careful and dispose of the spent match sensibly—dropping it down the toilet might cause blocked drains, and, remember, do not try this anywhere near a smoke detector.)

Traveling by Plane, Car, or Train

Traveling can be a frustrating experience if you have IBS. Even for healthy people, a trip takes planning, but traveling with a medical condition requires some special preparation for comfort. Don't be stuck at home because you're afraid to venture very far from a bathroom—learn how to travel without the stress.

Many public bathrooms on roadways or trains aren't clean or well stocked. Carry a little travel pack containing extra undergarments and trial sizes of toilet seat covers, wet wipes, antibacterial hand wash, extra toilet paper, and anything else you might need. If you need to go in a hurry, you can grab your bag and be off!

If you think it will help and it's feasible, pack a portable toilet. It might not be useful in urban areas, but when traveling off the beaten path it could be very helpful. When possible, arrange your meal schedule around your trip. If you know that you will have to use the toilet about an hour after a meal, be sure to leave enough time between your last meal and the start of the trip for a bathroom break. Make sure your traveling companions know that when you say you need to stop and find a bathroom, you mean *now*.

Flying causes a great deal of anxiety for many people, but you can minimize this anxiety by booking your ticket several weeks or even months before your trip. Ask for an aisle seat when you purchase your ticket. If you're comfortable doing so, ask for an aisle seat close to the plane's bathroom facilities.

Pack in your hand luggage extra undergarments, wet wipes, tissues, and any other items you might need in an emergency, or in the event a bathroom is not clean or well stocked. Also remember to pack a snack and some water—it's likely that you will not want to eat the food available in the airport or on the plane. Wear incontinence pants for an extra confidence boost.

If the airline does not give you an aisle seat, you can always politely ask another passenger to switch with you once everyone has boarded the plane. Passengers who won't mind switching seats with you might include someone who is traveling alone, a group traveling together that has been separated, or another passenger who wants the window seat.

Sex

IBS involves many issues, but it is not the easiest condition to have, especially for women, when it comes to the question of sex. Intercourse might be painful even when you are not having an attack, and if you are having an attack, sex is the last thing on your mind. You might even be afraid to get into a reclining position if you suffer from diarrhea, and if you have constipation, the last thing you want is someone on top of you.

The section on the next page entitled "Telling Other People" contains information that might be helpful when it comes to talking to your partner about your condition. This is really important when your partner wants to have sex and you do too, but your stomach doesn't. Your partner needs to understand that your digestive system is sensitive and that your sudden loss of libido has nothing to do with them and everything to do with the fact that you need to rush to the bathroom. If you do not want your partner to feel rejected and hurt, they have to know about your condition, know when to back off, and be willing to wait for a time that is more appropriate.

If your partner feels rejected because you seem to prefer the bathroom to them, then be sensitive to the hurt feelings involved and think about initiating sex when you feel better. Above all, do not use your IBS to avoid intimacy, or let IBS replace the "headache" excuse.

Painful Intercourse

Many women with IBS complain of a painful "crampy" feeling during sex. Because sex can be painful for many reasons, and several factors could be causing pain during sex apart from IBS, finding the solution can be a bit like solving a mystery (a very painful mystery).

First of all, it might help to try to work out when the pain started, how long you have had it, and where and when during intercourse you feel it.

Explore on your own. Exploring sexual pain yourself is particularly beneficial, because you don't have to worry about a partner poking you the wrong way. You can be as gentle as you want to be, and you're always in control.

Use plenty of lubrication. One of the most common reasons for painful sex is lack of lubrication. There are all sorts of reasons why women experience vaginal dryness (e.g., menopause), but using personal lubricant can be an easy and effective way to treat this problem and eliminate a major cause of painful sex.

Communicate with your partner. It can be difficult to talk about sex at the best of times, even for couples who have been together for many years. When it comes to talking about a difficult sexual issue, communication can get even trickier. But communication is the key to resolving painful sex. Even if the cause is entirely physical and will go away with treatment, it's still important to talk with your partner about the pain you're experiencing and work out other ways for both of you to satisfy your sexual needs while you are being treated for IBS.

Experiment with different sexual positions. For some people with IBS, pain during sex happens as a result of pressure on the abdomen. Try exploring different sexual positions and see if this alleviates some of the pain.

Consult your doctor or other health-care provider. If you can, in most cases it is worth talking with your doctor about this issue. Even if the problem clears up (or seems to clear up), pain during sex can be a symptom of other issues, and knowing this can alert your doctor to other questions that the doctor might want to ask.

Telling Other People

Keeping your condition a secret from the people you care about, and those who care about you, can lead to tension and misunderstandings, which will just make your symptoms worse, so it really is important that you talk about IBS.

Telling a partner or new friend (or even an old one) about your IBS condition is an embarrassing and personal subject that neither of you are likely to be comfortable with. But if you take time to think about whom, why, when, how, and where you will share your problems, it can bring you closer together.

Who? First of all decide if you really need to tell this person. Every acquaintance and business associate does not need to know. You'll want to know a new friend for at least a few months before sharing something so personal. This person should be trustworthy and be able to keep your condition confidential if you request it.

Why? Think about the reasons your friend needs to know about your IBS. Is it because you need to share with someone or because you want to become intimate? Perhaps you're spending a lot of time together, and your friend has noticed that you feel ill sometimes. Be honest with yourself about your reasons for communicating your issue.

How, when, and where? Once you decide to tell someone, make sure you talk in a quiet place where it's just the two of you, without distractions or other people who may interrupt. Start the conversation simply. Explain that you have health problems and the condition is chronic (it will come and go). There might be times when you are unable to attend events or have as much energy as others, but also explain that it does not mean you don't want to spend time with your friends or have fun. You want to live as normally as you can. You might also want to express to your friend that you are not asking them to "do" anything—except to be a good listener sometimes.

Only tell as much as you—and your friend—are comfortable with. You don't need to share every detail. If you're going to go on holiday with this person, they'll likely want to know about the "bathroom problems," but if it's a friend from work, for example, they might not want to know that you need to wear incontinence pants.

There's no doubt that it takes real courage to tell loved ones about your symptoms, but as Michael says below, the more that people can talk without embarrassment, the easier it will become for others to talk about it.

Michael, age 25

I still get embarrassed about my IBS, but I've crawled my way to a stage where I can mention it casually to my family and friends without any problems, and one day I hope to be able to say the word "constipation" aloud without turning purple.

If everyone with IBS tries not to be embarrassed, we're not only making things better for ourselves, we're making things better for all those who follow us. Every time someone talks about their bowel movements in public, it enables someone else to do the same—and if they're talking about it, they're on the way to finding help.

To the nonsufferers, I would ask you to consider your attitudes toward things like bathroom smells and flatulence. If your loved one has a terrible attack of diarrhea and stinks up the bathroom—so what? You love this person, don't you? Is it their fault? Are they really suffering? If you take a matter-of-fact attitude to bodily functions, smells, noises, and all the other nasty things we IBSers have to put up with, it will help your loved one realize that they are still loved and will help you both recognize that IBS does not define a person—it's the way you live that counts.

At work, talking to a trusted supervisor or coworker might make it easier for you to deal with your IBS condition. Let them know that you have a valid chronic illness, and when symptoms flare up, you have no control over it. This might mean bringing in educational materials, such as this book, to explain the condition. At the same time, tell this person that you've got a plan to deal with IBS, such as taking medication or going to the bathroom a few times a day, and that, despite it all, you are a dedicated worker.

You might well find that once you start telling people about your condition, most people will be more supportive if you're upfront with them. In fact, more people today know about IBS and understand its implications than ever before, and media awareness is increasing.

There are other sources of support if you don't feel comfortable talking with people you know. There are doctors, nurses, therapists, and dieticians who specialize in IBS and who can give you valuable feedback. You can also ask your doctor if he or she knows of any support groups. (The IBS Self Help and Support Group has meetings online at www.ibsgroup.org.)

Also, there are numerous websites for people with IBS. If you decide to log on and send an appeal or question to an online support group about something that worries you, you'll almost certainly get plenty of replies. Finding online support is easy. Just type the words "IBS support group" into your search engine and you'll find dozens of websites. Do be careful about buying products or following any medical advice advised on these websites, though, as they might not be medically approved. If you do hear about a treatment that has worked wonders for someone, as Jo did below, make sure you check it out with your doctor first.

Jo, age 37

I have suffered from IBS since I was about fifteen. I am now thirty-seven. At first I could cope with it because it was just occasional diarrhea, but over the years it has gotten worse and worse. I had all the usual tests done by the doctors, like everyone with IBS has had, and I was eventually told it was IBS and I would have to live with it.

I tried many prescription medications to no avail. I also went down the alternative route, but again with no luck. It was ruining my life. I couldn't go anywhere without knowing there was a bathroom nearby. My friends used to get fed up with me because I was always running off to the bathroom on shopping and theater outings. I have been caught short a number of times while out walking my dog (thank God for bushes!). I have even lost control in the kitchen of my house in front of my teenage son. I was absolutely mortified and cried and cried.

My savior was an IBS support group I found on the Internet. First, reading all about others with the condition and how much worse some are than me—and I thought I was bad enough—made me count my blessings a bit. Secondly, I heard about taking calcium for my IBS. I asked my doctor if it was worth a try, and he said it certainly was, so I tried it. Within two days this little (well big, actually) tablet completely changed my life. I no longer have diarrhea; it has been three months now and not once have I had it. I go once a day now, usually in the mornings, and it is completely normal, a normal shape, size, and color! I still can't believe it; really, I feel like a normal person. I no longer get the spasms, the bloating, the sickness—no symptoms whatsoever.

If, after reading this chapter, you still feel nervous about leaving the house for long periods of time, having a social life, or telling friends and loved ones about your symptoms, take things slowly at first. Invite people to your home, tell just one close friend, visit an IBS support group on the Web, and go out of the house for short periods of time. The cinema might be a bit too long for an outing, but a ten-minute short walk around the park certainly isn't. When you start to discover that you can survive these shorter outings, you will feel more confidence about getting out of the house more and gradually increasing the time you spend in public.

Helping Children and Teenagers Cope with IBS

Many people with IBS first develop symptoms during their teenage years or even during childhood. Symptoms like stomach pain, diarrhea, constipation, and bloating are difficult for adults to live with, but if you also have to cope with peer pressure, new relationships, new schools, puberty, and exams, it can make life very miserable indeed.

On top of this, teenagers often find that their parents, and even their doctors, do not take them seriously when they try to seek help. Stomachaches are often mistaken for anxiety about school work or other problems. This can be incredibly difficult for children, because not only do they have the physical pain and discomfort to deal with, they also have to get past the fact that everyone around them thinks they are "faking it."

Because of this problem, it is vital that parents pay attention when children or teenagers complain of problems "down there." Of course, most youngsters will try to get out of school once in a while, but very few will pretend to have such embarrassing symptoms as diarrhea or gas. In fact, it might take a great deal of courage for them to even admit to these symptoms in the first place. It's very important that when they do manage to talk about their problem, they receive a sympathetic ear.

If your child complains of stomach and bowel problems, it is vital that they receive a definite diagnosis of IBS from a doctor—bowel symptoms can mean IBS, but they can also mean a range of other disorders. Please get these ruled out before you assume that it's IBS. Once a diagnosis has been made, help your child find treatments that work for them. Many of the treatment approaches rec-ommended in *The IBS Healing Plan* will apply to your children as well, but it is important to work with the child's doctor.

It is also especially important that you tell your child that they are not to blame for the symptoms, and that IBS is not all in the mind. Having said this, stress and anxiety can be triggers for IBS, just as certain foods can be triggers for IBS, and so anything you can do to relieve stress might help relieve symptoms to a certain extent. Remember that your child might be worried about not reaching a bathroom in time and having an accident, or having to leave class during school time and being made fun of by the other children. At all stages of your child or teenager's illness, the best thing you can do is to support them and be there for them. If you are standing beside your child, saying IBS is real and it is miserable but that you are going to beat this together, then your child or teenager is much more likely to be hopeful and happy about the future, and your child will be far more willing to work with you to find the best treatment options.

Run, Don't Walk

It is helpful at this point for you to remind yourself of the top ten things you need to do to manage your IBS. Tear out or photocopy this page, or write down these points and pin them on your fridge or bathroom door—anywhere that you will be able to read them often:

1. Every human being passes gas and has bowel movements.

2. Your bowel is normal—just irritable.

3. Your bowel needs routine to stay healthy, so eat regularly and get enough sleep.

4. Keep a food diary to identify food triggers.

5. Eat enough (but not too much) fiber (25 to 30 grams a day) and drink six to eight glasses of water a day.

6. Practice stress-management techniques.

7. Get some fresh air and exercise every day.

8. One in five people have IBS—you are not alone.

9. Work with your doctor and talk about any concerns or fears you might have.

10. Take control of your IBS symptoms.

Above all, pay attention to point number ten: Take control of your IBS symptoms so that they don't control you. This book has given you the tools you need to take control. It's up to you, now, to discover what works best for your IBS so you can start living again and running, rather than walking, toward your dreams.

References

Chapter 1: What Is IBS?

Azpiroz, F., and M. Bouin. 2007. Mechanisms of hypersensitivity in IBS and functional disorders. *Neurogastroenterology Motility* 19(1 Suppl): 62–88.

Kolfenbach, L. 2007. Pathophysiology, diagnosis, and treatment of IBS. *Journal of the American Academy of Physician Assistants* 20(1): 16–20.

Talley, N. J. 2006. Irritable bowel syndrome. *International Medicine Journal* 36(11): 724–8.

Chapter 2: What Causes IBS?

Azpiroz, F., et al. 2000. Nongastrointestinal disorders in the irritable bowel syndrome. *Digestion* 62: 66–72.

Bengston, M. B. 2006. Irritable bowel syndrome in twins: genes and environment. *Gut* 55(12): 1754–9. Epub.

Blumental, M., et al., Editors. 2000. *Herbal Medicine: Expanded Commission E Monographs*, American Botanical Council with IntegrativMedicine Communications. Newton, MA: Lippincott Williams & Wilkins.

Case, A. M., and R. L. Reid. 1998. Effects of the menstrual cycle on medical disorders. *Archives of Internal Medicine* 158: 1405–12. http://www.ama-assn.org/special/womh/library/readroom/arch98/ira70759.htm.

Eliakim, R., et al. 2000. Progesterone and the gastrointestinal tract. *The Journal of Reproductive Medicine* 45(10): 781–8.

Ewaschuk, J. B., et al. 2006. The role of antibiotic and probiotic therapies in current and future management of inflammatory bowel disease. *Current Gastroenterology Reports* 8(6): 486–98.

Fanigliulo, F. 2006. Role of gut microflora and probiotic effects in the irritable bowel syndrome. *Acta Biomedica* 77(2): 85–9.

Garrigues, V., et al. 2007. Change over time of bowel habit in irritable bowel syndrome: A prospective, observational, 1-year follow-up study (RITMO study). *Alimentary Pharmacology and Therapeutics* 25(3): 323–32. Epub.

Gilbody, J. S., et al. 2000. Comparison of two different formulations of mebeverine hydrochloride in irritable bowel syndrome. *International Journal of Clinical Practice* 54(7): 461–4.

Jones, J., et al. 2000. British Society of Gastroenterology guidelines for the management of irritable bowel syndrome. *Gut* (Suppl II), 47: 1–19.

Khosh, F. 2000. A natural approach to irritable bowel syndrome. *Townsend Letter for Doctors and Patients* 7:62–4.

Locke, G. R., et al. 2000. Risk factors for irritable bowel syndrome: role of analgesics and food sensitivities. *American Journal of Gastroenterology* 95(1): 157–65.

Olesen, M., and E. Gudmund-Hoyer. 2000. Efficacy, safety, and tolerability of fructooligosaccharides in the treatment of irritable bowel syndrome. *American Journal of Clinical Nutrition* 72:1570–5.

Oxol, D. 2006. Relationship between asthma and irritable bowel syndrome: Role of food allergy. *Journal of Asthma* 43(10): 773–5.

Playford, R. J., et al. 1999. Bovine colostrum is a health food supplement which prevents NSAID-induced gut damage. *Gut* 44:653–8.

Quigley, E. M., et al. 2007. Bacterial flora in irritable bowel syndrome: Role in pathophysiology, implications for management. *Chinese Journal of Digestive Diseases* 8(1): 2–7.

Sanger, G. J. 1996. 5-Hydroxytryptamine and functional bowel disorders. *Neurogastroenterology Motility* 8:319–31.

Shaheen, S. O., et al. 2000. Frequent paracetamol use and asthma in adults. *Thorax* 55:266–70.

Spiller, R. C. 2007. Role of infection in irritable bowel syndrome. *Journal of Gastroenterology* 42(Suppl, 17): 41–7.

Tamboli, C. P., et al. 2004. Dysbiosis in inflammatory bowel disease. *Gut* 53(1): 1–4.

Varner, A. E., Reply to Locke et al. 2000. Risk factors for irritable bowel syndrome. *American Journal of Gastroenterology*, p. 3310.

Chapter 3: Do You Have IBS?

Chang, F. Y. 2007. Irritable bowel syndrome in the 21st century: Perspectives from Asia or South-east Asia. *Journal of Gastroenterology and Hepatology* 22(1): 4–12.

Garrigues, V., et al. 2007. Change over time of bowel habit in irritable bowel syndrome: A prospective, observational, 1-year follow-up study

(RITMO study). *Alimentary Pharmacology and Therapeutics* 1, 25(3): 323–32. Epub.

Kajander, K. 2006. Clinical studies on alleviating the symptoms of irritable bowel syndrome. *Asia Pacific Journal of Clinical Nutrition* 15(4): 576–80.

Kolfenbach, L. et al. 2007. Pathophysiology, diagnosis, and treatment of IBS. *Journal of the American Academy of Physicians* 20(1): 16–20.

Spinelli, A. 2007. Irritable bowel syndrome. *Clinical Drug Investigation* 27(1): 15–33.

Chapter 4: Healing IBS with Diet

Bijkerk, C. J., et al. 2004. Systematic review: the role of different types of fiber in the treatment of irritable bowel syndrome. *Alimentary Pharmacology and Therapeutics* 1, 19(3): 245–51. Review.

Bolin, T. D. 2005. Irritable bowel syndrome. *Australian Family Physician* 34(4): 221–4.

Dapoigny, M., et al. 2003. Role of alimentation in irritable bowel syndrome. *Digestion* 67(4): 225–33.

Drisko, J. 2006. Treating irritable bowel syndrome with a food elimination diet followed by food challenge and probiotics. *Journal of the American College of Nutrition* 25(6): 514–22.

Farthing, M. J. 2004. Treatment options in irritable bowel syndrome. *Best Practice and Research Clinical Gastroenterology* 18(4): 773–86.

Goldstein, R., et al. 2000. Carbohydrate malabsorption and the effect of dietary restriction on symptoms of irritable bowel syndrome and functional bowel complaints. *Israel Medical Association Journal* 2(8): 583–7.

Macdermott, R. P. 2007. Treatment of irritable bowel syndrome in outpatients with inflammatory bowel disease using a food and beverage intolerance, food and beverage avoidance diet. *Inflammatory Bowel Disorders* 13(1): 91–6.

Watson, A. R., and T. E. Bowling. 2005. Irritable bowel syndrome: diagnosis and symptom management. *British Journal of Community Nursing* 10(3): 118–22.

Joung, Kim Y., and D. J. Ban. 2005. Prevalence of irritable bowel syndrome, influence of lifestyle factors and bowel habits in Korean college students. *International Journal Nursing Students* 42(3): 247–54.

Kanazawa, M., and S. Fukudo. 2006. Effects of fasting therapy on irritable bowel syndrome. *International Journal of Behavioral Medicine* 13(3): 214–20.

Chapter 5: Healing IBS with Supplements

Akobeng, A. K., et al. 2000. Double-blind randomized controlled trial of glutamine-enriched polymeric diet in the treatment of active Crohn's disease. *Journal of Pediatric Gastroenterology and Nutrition* 30(1): 78–84.

Aller, R., et al. 2004. Dietary intake of a group of patients with irritable bowel syndrome: Relation between dietary fiber and symptoms. *Anales de Medicina Interna* 21(12): 577–80.

Aquino, R., et al. 1989. Plant metabolites. Structure and in vitro antiviral activity of quinovic acid glycosides from Uncaria tomentosa and Guettarda platypoda. *Journal of Natural Products* 52(4): 679–85.

Aquino, R., et al. 1990. New polyhydroxylated triterpenes from Uncaria tomentosa. *Journal of Natural Products* 53(3): 559–64.

Aquino R., et al. 1981. Plant metabolites: New compounds and anti-inflammatory activity of Uncaria tomentosa. *Journal of Natural Products* 54(2): 453–9.

Arimi, S. M. 1989. Campylobacter infection in humans. *East African Medical Journal* 66(12): 851–5.

Aziz, N. H. 1998. Comparative antibacterial and antifungal effects of some phenolic compounds. *Microbios* 93(374): 43–54.

Beesley, A., et al. 1996. Influence of peppermint oil on absorptive and secretory processes in rat small intestine. *Gut* 39(2): 214–19.

Cavallo, G., et al. 1990. Changes in the blood zinc in the irritable bowel syndrome: A preliminary study. *Minerva Dietol Gastroenterol* 36(2): 77–81.

Chang, H. Y., et al. 2006. Current gut-directed therapies for irritable bowel syndrome. *Current Treatment Options Gastroenterology* 9(4): 314–23.

Chapman, N. D., et al. 1990. A comparison of mebeverine with high-fiber dietary advice and mebeverine plus ispaghula in the treatment of irritable bowel syndrome: An open, prospectively randomised, parallel group study. *British Journal of Clinical Practice* 44(11): 461.

Fernandez-Banares, F., et al. 1999. Randomized clinical trial of Plantago ovata seeds (dietary fiber) as compared with mesalamine in maintaining remission in ulcerative colitis, Spanish Group for the Study of Crohn's Disease and Ulcerative Colitis (GETECCU). *American Journal of Gastroenterology* 94(2): 427–33.

Fujita, T., and K. Sakurai. 1995. Efficacy of glutamine-enriched enteral nutrition in an experimental model of mucosal ulcerative colitis. *British Journal of Surgery* 82:749–51.

Grigoleit, H. 2005. Pharmacology and preclinical pharmacokinetics of peppermint oil. *Phytomedicine* 12(8): 612–16.

Hotz, J., et al. 1994. Effectiveness of plantago seed husks in comparison with wheat bran on stool frequency and manifestations of irritable colon syndrome with constipation. *Medical Klin* 89(12): 645–51.

Ionescu, G., et al. 1990. Oral citrus seed extract. *Journal of Orthomolecular Medicine* 5(3): 72–4.

Jones, K. 1995. *Cat's Claw: Healing Vine of Peru*. Seattle, WA: Sylvan Press, pp. 48–9.

Liu, J. H., et al. 1997. Enteric-coated peppermint-oil capsules in the treatment of irritable bowel syndrome: A prospective, randomized trial. *Journal of Gastroenterology* 32(6): 765–8.

MacMahon, M., et al. 1998. Ispaghula husk in the treatment of hypercholesterolaemia: A double-blind controlled study. *Journal of Cardiovascular Risk* 5(3): 167–72.

McKay, D. L., and J. B. Blumberg. 2006. A review of the bioactivity and potential health benefits of peppermint tea (Mentha piperita L.). *Phytotherapy Research* 20(8): 619–33.

Nash, P., et al. 1986. Peppermint oil does not relieve the pain of irritable bowel syndrome. *British Journal of Clinical Practice* 40(7): 292–3.

Nobaek, S., et al. 2000. Alteration of intestinal microflora is associated with reduction in abdominal bloating and pain in patients with irritable bowel syndrome. *American Journal of Gastroenterology* 95(5): 1231–8.

Pittler, M. H. 1998. Peppermint oil for irritable bowel syndrome: A critical review and metaanalysis. *American Journal of Gastroenterology* 93(7): 1131–5.

Quigley, E. M., et al. 2007. Probiotics and irritable bowel syndrome: A rationale for their use and an assessment of the evidence to-date. *Neurogastroenterol Motility* 19(3): 166–72.

Rees, W. D. 1979. Treating irritable bowel syndrome with peppermint oil. *British Medical Journal* 2(6194): 835–6.

Sandoval-Chacon, M. 1998. Antiinflammatory actions of cat's claw: The role of NF-kappaB. *Aliment Pharmacology and Therapeutics* 12(12): 1279–89.

Shulz, V., et al. 1996. *Rational Phythotherapy: A Physician's Guide to Herbal Medicine.* New York: Springer-Verlag, pp. 187–90.

Simmen, U., et al. 2006. Binding of STW 5 (Iberogast(R)) and its components to intestinal 5-HT, muscarinic M(3), and opioid receptors. *Phytomedicine* 13 (Suppl 1): 51–5), Epub.

Tassou, C. C. 1991. Effect of phenolic compounds and oleuropein on the germination of Bacillus cereus T spores. *Biotechnology and Applied Biochemistry* 13(2): 231–7.

Tomas-Ridocci, M., et al. 1992. The efficacy of Plantago ovata as a regulator of intestinal transit, (A double-blind study compared to placebo). *Rev Esp Enferm Dig* 82(1): 17–22.

Torri, A., et al. 2004. Management of irritable bowel syndrome. *Internal Medicine* 43(5): 353–9.

Valberg, L. S., et al. 1986. Zinc absorption in inflammatory bowel disease. *Digestive Diseases and Sciences* 31(7): 724–31.

Visioli, F., et al. 1998. Oleuropein, the bitter principle of olives, enhances nitric oxide production by mouse macrophages. *Life Sciences* 62(6): 541–6.

Walker, A. F., et al. 2001. Artichoke leaf extract reduces symptoms of irritable bowel syndrome in a post-marketing surveillance study. *Phytotherapy Research* 15(1): 58–61.

Wong, P. W., et al. 1999. How to deal with chronic constipation. A stepwise method of establishing and treating the source of the problem. *Postgraduate Medicine* 106(6): 199–200, 203–4, 207–10.

Chapter 6: Healing IBS with Complementary Therapies

Bensoussan, A. 2001. Establishing evidence for Chinese medicine: A case example of irritable bowel syndrome. *Zhonghua Yi Xue Za Zhi (Taipei)* 64(9): 487–92.

Carmona-Sanchez, R., and F. A. Tostado-Fernandez. 2005. Prevalence of use of alternative and complementary medicine in patients with irritable bowel syndrome, functional dyspepsia and gastresophageal reflux disease. *Revista de Gastroenterología de México* 70(4): 393–8.

Chan, J., et al. 1997. The role of acupuncture in the treatment of irritable bowel syndrome: A pilot study. *Hepatogastroenterology* 44:1328–30.

Fireman, Z., et al. 2001. Acupuncture treatment for irritable bowel syndrome. A double-blind controlled study. *Digestion* 64:100–3.

Galovski, T. E., and E. B. Blanchard. 1998. The treatment of irritable bowel syndrome with hypnotherapy. *Applied Psychophysiology and Biofeedback* 23:219–32.

Gholamrezaei, A., et al. 2006. Where does hypnotherapy stand in the management of irritable bowel syndrome? *Journal of Alternative and Complementary Medicine* 12(6): 517–27.

Harvey, R. F., et al. 1989. Individual and group hypnotherapy in treatment of refractory irritable bowel syndrome. *Lancet* 1:424–5.

Houghton, L. A., et al. 1996. Symptomatology, quality of life and economic features of irritable bowel syndrome—the effect of hypnotherapy. *Alimentary Pharmacology Therapeutics* 10:91–5.

Keefer, L., and E. B. Blanchard. 2002. A one year follow-up of relaxation response meditation as a treatment for irritable bowel syndrome. *Behaviour Research Therapy* 40:541–6.

Lim, B., et al. 2006. Acupuncture for treatment of irritable bowel syndrome. *Cochrane Database Syst Rev* 18(4).

Spanier, J. A., et al. 2003. A systematic review of alternative therapies in the irritable bowel syndrome. *Archives of Internal Medicine* 163: 265–74.

Chapter 7: Healing IBS with Stress Management

Gupta, N. 2006. Effect of yoga based lifestyle intervention on state and trait anxiety. *Indian Journal of Physiology and Pharmacology* 50(1): 41–7.

Keefer, L., and E. B. Blanchard. 2002. Related articles, a one year follow-up of relaxation response meditation as a treatment for irritable bowel syndrome. *Behavioral Research Therapy* 40(5): 541–6.

Levy, R. L., et al. 2005. The association of gastrointestinal symptoms with weight, diet, and exercise in weight-loss program participants. *Clinical Gastroenterology and Hepatology* 3(10): 992–6.

Lustyk, M. K., et al. 2001. Does a physically active lifestyle improve symptoms in women with irritable bowel syndrome? *Gastroenterology Nursing* 24(3): 129–37.

Orr, W. C. 2001. Gastrointestinal functioning during sleep: A new horizon in sleep medicine. *Sleep Medicine Reviews* 5(2): 91–101.

Toner, B. B. 2005. Cognitive-behavioral treatment of irritable bowel syndrome. *CNS Spectrums* 10(11): 883–90.

Villoria, A., et al. 2006. Physical activity and intestinal gas clearance in patients with bloating. *American Journal of Gastroenterology* 101(11): 2552–7. Epub.

Whitehead, W. E., et al. 1992. Effects of stressful life events on bowel symptoms: Subjects with irritable bowel syndrome compared with subjects without bowel dysfunction. *Gut* 33(6): 825–30.

Chapter 8: Working with Your Doctor

Chang, H. Y. 2006. Current gut-directed therapies for irritable bowel syndrome. *Current Treatment Options Gastroenterology* 9(4): 314–23.

Dellon, E. S., et al. 2006. Treatment of functional diarrhea, *Current Treatment Options Gastroenterology* 9(4): 331–42.

Klein, K. B. 1988. Controlled treatment trials in the irritable bowel syndrome: A critique. *Gastroenterology* 95:232–41.

Lacy, B. E. 2005. Irritable bowel syndrome: A syndrome in evolution. *Journal of Clinical Gastroenterology* 39(5 Suppl): S230–42.

Quartero, A. O., et al. 2005. Bulking agents, antispasmodic and antidepressant medication for the treatment of irritable bowel syndrome. *Cochrane Database System Reviews* 18(2).

Tillisch, K. 2005. Diagnosis and treatment of irritable bowel syndrome: State of the art. *Current Gastroenterology Reports* 7(4): 249–56.

Chapter 9: A-to-Z of Specific Symptoms and Natural Ways to Beat Them

Carmona-Sanchez, R., et al. 2005. Prevalence of use of alternative and complementary medicine in patients with irritable bowel syndrome, functional dyspepsia and gastresophageal reflux disease. *Rev Gastroenterology Mexico* 70(4): 393–8.

Cremonini, F., and N. J. Talley. Diagnostic and therapeutic strategies in the irritable bowel syndrome. *Minerva Medicine* 95(5): 427–41.

Dellon, E. S., and Y. Ringel. 2006. Treatment of functional diarrhea. *Current Treatment Options Gastroenterology* 9(4): 331–42.

Fernandez-Banares, F. 2006. Nutritional care of the patient with constipation. *Best Practice and Research Clinical Gastroenterology* 20(3): 575–87.

Gerson, M. J., et al. 2005. An international study of irritable bowel syndrome: Family relationships and mind-body attributions. *Social Science and Medicine* 62(11): 2838–47. Epub.

Kim, H. J., et al. 2005. A randomized controlled trial of a probiotic combination VSL# 3 and placebo in irritable bowel syndrome with bloating. *Neurogastroenterology Motility* 17(5): 687–96.

McKay, D. L., and J. B. Blumberg. 2006. A review of the bioactivity and potential health benefits of peppermint tea (Mentha piperita L.). *Phytotherapy Research* 20(8): 619–33.

Torii, A., and G. Toda. 2004. Management of irritable bowel syndrome. *Internal Medicine* 43(5): 353–9.

Chapter 10: Living with IBS

Amouretti, M., et al. 2006. Impact of irritable bowel syndrome (IBS) on health-related quality of life (HRQOL). *Gastroenterology Clinical Biol* 30(2): 241–6.

Authors unknown. 2006. Is there any food I can eat? Living with inflammatory bowel disease and/or irritable bowel syndrome. *Clinical Nurse Specialist* 20(5): 241–7.

Chiba, T., et al. 2006. Quality of life in irritable bowel syndrome. *Nippon Rinsho* 64(8): 1540–3.

Smith, G. D. 2006. Irritable bowel syndrome: Quality of life and nursing interventions. *British Journal of Nursing* 15(21): 1152–6.

Varni, J. W., et al. 2006. Health-related quality of life in pediatric patients with irritable bowel syndrome: A comparative analysis. *Journal of Developmental and Behavioral Pediatrics* 27(6): 451–8.

Resources

If you suffer from IBS, there are many resources that offer support, help, and advice. In this section you'll find support groups, websites, and books that can help you learn more about the condition and put you in touch with other people who also have IBS.

USA

IBS Association (IBSA)
Address as IBS Self Help Group (below)
E-mail: ibsa@ibsassociation.org
Website: www.ibsassociation.org
A nonprofit organization offering support groups, information, and education.

IBS Self Help Group (IBS Group)
1440 Whalley Ave., #145
New Haven CT 06515
E-mail: ibs@ibsgroup.org
Website: www.ibsgroup.org

International Foundation for Functional Digestive Disorders (IFFGD)
PO Box 170864
Milwaukee W1 53217-806
(414) 964-1799
E-mail: iffgd@iffgd.org
Website: www.iffgd.org
A nonprofit organization dedicated to education and research.

Canada

IBS Self-Help and Support Group (IBS Group)
PO Box 94074
Toronto, Ontario MN4 3R1
E-mail: ibs@ibsgroup.org
Website: www.ibsgroup.org

The Canadian Society of Intestinal Research
855 West 12th Ave.
Vancouver, British Columbia V5Z 1M9
(604) 875-4875
Website: www.badgut.com
Offers information, live support groups, and online support.

Australia

IBIS Australia
PO Box 7092
Sippy Downs
Qld 7092
Phone: 1300 651 131
E-mail: contact@ibis-australia.org
Website: www.ibs-australia.org

Self-Help Websites

www.helpforibs.com
Help for IBS is a site owned by IBS sufferer and expert Heather Van Horous. It provides information, education, recipes, and IBS-related products. You can also sign up for online support groups and message boards.

www.ibsgroup.org
This IBS self-help and support group claims to be the largest online patient advocate and support community for people with IBS.

www.ibstales.com
IBS Tales is a site where people with IBS can tell their stories and read about the experiences of others.

E-mail Lists

If you join a mailing list server, you can receive e-mails from people who also have IBS. These lists provide the opportunity to communicate about IBS with others who have the condition. For example, the following are both general lists that are dedicated to IBS discussion:

health.groups.yahoo.com/group/irritable-bowel-syndrome

http://health.groups.yahoo.com/group/ibspag

Further Reading

Bolen, Barbara, and Jeffrey Roberts. *IBS Chat: Real Life Stories and Solutions*. Lincoln, NE: iUniverse, Inc., 2007.

Braimbridge, Sophie, and Erica Jankovich. *Healthy Eating for IBS*. London: Kyle Cathie, 2005.

Brewer, Sarah, and Michelle Berriedale-Johnson. *IBS Diet: Reduce Pain and Improve Digestion the Natural Way*. London: Thorson's, 2004.

Burstall, Dawn. *IBS Relief: A Complete Approach to Managing Irritable Bowel Syndrome*. Hoboken, NJ: John Wiley, 2006.

Dean, Carolyn, and Christine Wheeler. *IBS for Dummies*. Hoboken, NJ: For Dummies, 2005.

Farhadi, Ashkan. *I Have IBS...Now What?!!! A Comprehensive Guide for Patients with Irritable Bowel Syndrome*. Charleston, SC: BookSurge Publishing, 2007.

Nicol, Rosemary. *The Irritable Bowel Diet Book*. London: Sheldon Press, 1991.

Smith, Tom. *Coping with Heartburn and Reflux*. London: Sheldon Press, 2006.

Van Vorous, Heather. *Eating for IBS: 175 Delicious, Nutritious, Low-Fat, Low-Residue Recipes to Stabilize the Touchiest Tummy*. New York: Marlowe & Company, 2000.

Van Vorous, Heather. *The First Year: IBS (Irritable Bowel Syndrome)—An Essential Guide for the Newly Diagnosed (Patient-Expert Guides)*. New York: Marlowe & Company, 2005.

Index

A

abdominal massage, 78
abdominal pain: easing, 101–102; recurring bouts of, 19
abdominal swelling, 20
abdominal training, 76
abdominal windmills, 76
acetaminophen, 13, 101–102
acetylcholine, 13
acupressure, 57, 128
acupuncture, 57, 60
adrenaline production, 68
age, 21
alcohol, 32–33, 89; eating out and, 40
ALE. *See* artichoke leaf extract
American Journal of Clinical Hypnosis, 61
American Journal of Gastroenterology, 72
amino acids, 26
analgesics, 13
anise, 49, 127
antidepressants, 94–95
antispasmodics, 95
anxiety, 102–105; food and, 105; gas and, 122
apples, 126
aromatherapy, 58–59, 86; bloating and, 108; fatigue and, 121; headaches and, 125
artichoke, 116
artichoke leaf extract (ALE), 49
avocados, 90
Ayurveda, 85–86

B

bach flower remedies, 115
bacteria overgrowth, 15
baking soda, 126
bananas, 90, 107, 118
baths, 104
beans, 109
behavioral therapy, 70–72; cognitive, 71
biofeedback, 71
bloating, 20, 105–108; aromatherapy and, 108; cause of, 106, 108; food alleviating, 107
blood sugar, 103
blueberries, 117–118
bowel, large, 8–9
bowel movements: abnormal, 19–20; change in, 20; incomplete emptying sensation after, 20
bowel, small, 8
breathing, 69–70; exercises, 82; meditation, 79; relaxation therapy, 82; stress release and, 69–70; yoga and, 62
briefs, adult, 131

C

caffeine, 106, 119; headaches and, 124
cake, 32
calcium, 46, 112; channel blocker, 52
Calmactin, 97
caraway, 49
carbohydrates, 25–26; complex, 25; fatigue and, 120; refined, 26; unrefined, 26

carbonation, 33
catnip, 103
cat's claw, 49–50
challenges, 114
chamomile, 50, 87, 103, 128; tea, 118
children, 138–139
Chinese medicine, traditional (TCM), 59–60, 115
chocolate, 32
cinnamon, 127
co-enzyme Q10, 121
coffee, 31, 89
colonic massage, 111, 119
constipation, 108–111; fiber and, 109; yoga for, 62–63
corticotrophin-releasing factor (CRF), 15
counseling, 72
CRF. *See* corticotrophin-releasing factor
cumin, 127
cycling, 75

D

dairy products, 12, 30, 46
daydreaming, 85
de-cluttering, 86
depression, 113–117; food and, 116–117; fruit and, 116; water and, 117
diapers, adult, 130
diarrhea, 117–120; diarrhea-predominant irritable bowel syndrome, 13; doctors and, 120; fruit and, 117–118; yoga for, 63
diet, 38–39; adjusting, 27–39; healthy, 24–25; journal, 28–29; menstrual cycle and, 112; pain from, 23; plan, 39; rules of, seven golden, 39–40; trigger, 29–33; vegetarian, 41–42
digestive aids, 52–54
doctors, 93; diarrhea and, 120; visiting, 97–98
drugs, 21–22, 93, 99; acetaminophen, 13, 101–102; antidepressant, 94–95; antispasmodic, 95; Calmactin, 97;

Imodium, 96; irritable bowel syndrome and, 21–22; Lomotil, 96; Lotronex, 95–96; narcotics, 96–97; over-the-counter, 93–94; prescription, 94–97; Zelnorm, 97

E

eating out, 40–41; alcohol and, 40; appetizers and, 41; awkward questions and, 41; bathrooms and, 40
EFAs. *See* essential fatty acids
EPO. *See* evening primrose oil
esophagus, symptoms relating to, 8
essential fatty acids (EFAs), 33–34
evening primrose oil (EPO), 50
exercise, 72–77, 89, 114; abdominal training, 76; abdominal windmill, 76; bloating and, 106; cycling as, 75; dressing for, 77; entertainment during, 77; fatigue and, 120; getting started with, 73–74; jogging as, 75; journal, 77; menstrual cycle and, 113; partners, 76; relaxation, 80–82; sample plan for, 74–75; scheduling, 77; stomach contraction, 76; swimming as, 75; toning, 75–76; trampoline as, 75; visualization, 82–84; walking as, 74–75

F

fatigue, 120–121; aromatherapy and, 121; carbohydrates and, 120; co-enzyme Q10 and, 121; exercise and, 120; ginger and, 121
fats, 27; artificial, 33; healthy, 33–34; saturated, 30–31
fecal incontinence, 130–131
fennel, 50–51, 127; tea, 107
fiber, 24, 107; constipation and, 109; insoluble, 35–37; intake, 37–38; soluble, 34–35, 36, 38, 53–54
fish, 34, 105, 117; depression and, 117
5-HIAA, 13
food: antianxiety, 105; bloating and, 107; depression and, 116–117;

fluid retention, 106; selenium-rich, 105; zinc-rich, 105. *See also specific foods*
food intolerance, 12
fruits, 32, 90; constipation and, 109–110; depression and, 116; diarrhea and, 117–118; problem, 36–37. *See also specific fruits*
functional disorder, 6

G
games, mind, 90–91
gamma-linolenic acid (GLA), 50
garlic, 110
gas, 121–123; anxiety and, 122; smoking and, 122; yoga for, 63–64
gastrointestinal contractions, 6
gastrointestinal system (GI), 6; irritants, 31–33
genetics, 12
GI. *See* gastrointestinal system
ginger, 51, 115, 128; fatigue and, 121; tea, 123
GLA. *See* gamma-linolenic acid
glucose, 25
grains, 12
grape, Oregon, 109
grapefruit, 116
grapefruit seed, 51
gum, chewing, 33
gut dysbiosis, 16–17

H
headaches, 124–126; aromatherapy and, 125; magnesium and, 124; massage and, 125; triggers, 124
heartburn, 126–127; herbs for, 127; massage for, 126; triggers, 126
heat, therapeutic, 58
herbal healing, 49–52, 103; for heartburn, 127
homeopathy, 60–61
honey, 110
hot water with lemon, 110
hypnotherapy, 61–62, 71

I
IBS. *See* irritable bowel syndrome
IFFGD. *See* International Foundation for Functional Gastrointestinal Disorders
Imodium, 96
indigestion, yoga for, 64–65
International Foundation for Functional Gastrointestinal Disorders (IFFGD), 7
intestine, small, 15
irritable bowel syndrome (IBS): age and, 21; cause of, 11–12; cause of, eating-related, 24–25; children and, 138–139; confusion over, 22; diagnosing, 7; diarrhea-predominant, 13; drugs and, 21–22; early warning signs, 17–18; food intolerance and, 12; inheritance of, 12; managing, 139–140; mood and, 14–15; origins of, 11; perception of, 113; questionnaire, 19–21; statistics of, key, 22; stress and, 22; symptoms of, 2, 7–10, 19–21; symptoms of, clinical, 111–113; symptoms of, most common, 9; symptoms of, nonbowel, 21; teenagers and, 138–139; testing for, 6; triggering, 22, 29–33; women and, 111–113

J
jogging, 75

L
large bowel, 8–9
lavender oil, 90
laxatives, 108
leaky gut syndrome, 16–17; diet and, 17; stress and, 17
lemon balm, 103
lentils, 117
L-glutamine, 118–119
LH. *See* luteinizing hormone
lime juice, 127
Lomotil, 96

Lotronex, 95–96
luteinizing hormone (LH), 14

M
magnesium, 46–47, 112; headaches
   and, 124
massage, 77–78, 115; abdominal, 78;
   colonic, 111, 119; foot, 66–67; headaches and, 125; for heartburn, 126;
   shiatsu, 57
meat, red, 30
meditation, 78–79; breathing, 79; gaz-
   ing, 79; mantra, 78; relaxation-
   response, 62; walking, 79
menstrual cycle, 13–14; diet and, 112;
   exercise and, 113; IBS and, 111–113
meridians, 57
mint, 128
molasses, blackstrap, 109
monosodium glutamate (MSG), 33
motherwort, 103
movement therapy, 62–67
MSG. See monosodium glutamate
mucous colitis. See irritable bowel syndrome
mucus, 20
music therapy, 79–80, 104

N
narcotics, 96–97
nature v. nurture, 12
nausea, 127–128
nerve function, 13
neurochemical imbalances, 12–13
norepinephrine, 12–13
nutrient deficiency, 17

O
oatmeal, 32
odors, covering up, 131
oil: carrier, 58; essential, 58–59, 104;
   lavender, 90; olive, 107; peppermint,
   52; safflower, 110; soybean, 110;
   vegetable, 110
olive leaf, 51

onion, 127
optimism, 104
orange peel, 118
oregano, 51

P
pain: abdominal, 19, 101–102; from
   diet, 23; perception, 6; sex and,
   133–134
panty liners, 130
passionflower, 103
peppermint oil, 52
personal space, 84–85
pet, stroking your, 87
posture, 115–116
potatoes, 118
probiotics, 53
progesterone, 13
prostaglandins E2/F2 alpha, 14, 33
protein, 26
psychotherapy, traditional, 71–72
psyllium, 53–54, 108

Q
Qi, 57
questionnaire, IBS, 19–21

R
reflexology, 65–67
Reiki, 80
relaxation therapy, 71, 80–82, 104;
   back, 82; biceps, 81; breath, 82; but-
   tock, 82; calf, 82; eye, 81–82; foot,
   82; hand, 81; mouth, 81; neck, 81;
   shoulder, 81; stomach, 82; thigh, 82;
   toe, 82; tongue, 81; triceps, 81
reproductive hormones, 13–14
restaurants. See eating out

S
safety, 100–101
Saint John's wort, 114–115
salt, 105
serotonin, 12–13; 5-HT3 receptor, 13;
   imbalance in, 13

sesame seeds, 110
sex, 90, 132–134; communication regarding, 134; painful, 133–134
shiatsu massage, 57
sleep, 87–91
small bowel, 8
smoking, 89; gas and, 122
space, personal, 84–85
spastic colon. *See* irritable bowel syndrome
starches, 34
stomach: noises, 123–124; symptoms relating to, 8
stomach contractions, 76
stress, 14–15, 68–69; irritable bowel syndrome and, 22; leaky gut syndrome and, 17
sunflower seeds, 116
sunlight, 115
supplements, mineral, 45–47, 48–49
supplements, vitamin, 47–49; A, 48; B, 105, 106; D, 48; E, 48; K, 48
sweeteners, artificial, 33
sweets, 32
swimming, 75

T

TCM. *See* Chinese medicine, traditional
tea, 89; chamomile, 118; fennel, 107; ginger, 123
teenagers, 138–139
testosterone, 14
therapeutic heat, 58

toilet, portable, 132
toning exercises, 75–76
trampoline, 75
traveling, 131–132
twins, identical, 12

V

valerian root, 85, 103
vegetables: problem, 36–37. *See also specific vegetables*
vegetarianism, 41–42
vinegar, 110
visualization exercises, 82–84
Vitex agnus-castus, 112–113

W

walking, 74–75
walnuts, 109
warning signs, early, 17–18
water, 26–27; depression and, 117
watermelon, 116
weight loss, 42–43
women: IBS and, 111–113
writing, 87

Y

yoga, 103–104; breath and, 62; constipation, 62–63; diarrhea and, 63; gas and, 63–64; indigestion and, 65
yogurt, soy, 107

Z

Zelnorm, 97
zinc, 47; rich food, 105